THE GHOST WILL SEE YOU NOW

Books by Randy Russell

Ghost Story Collections

Ghost Cats of the South
Ghost Dogs of the South (with Janet Barnett)
The Granny Curse and Other Ghosts and Legends from East Tennessee
  (with Janet Barnett)
Mountain Ghost Stories and Curious Tales of Western North Carolina
  (with Janet Barnett)

Novels

Dead Rules
Doll Eyes
Caught Looking
Blind Spot
Hot Wire

THE GHOST WILL SEE YOU NOW

HAUNTED HOSPITALS OF THE SOUTH

by
Randy
Russell

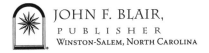
JOHN F. BLAIR,
PUBLISHER
WINSTON-SALEM, NORTH CAROLINA

JOHN F. BLAIR,
PUBLISHER

1406 Plaza Drive
Winston-Salem, North Carolina 27103
www.blairpub.com

Library of Congress Cataloging-in-Publication Data

Russell, Randy.
  The ghost will see you now : haunted hospitals of the south / by Randy Russell.
    pages   cm
  ISBN 978-0-89587-631-7 (alk. paper) — ISBN 978-0-89587-632-4 (ebook) 1.
Haunted hospitals—Southern States. I. Title.
  BF1474.4.R87 2014
  133.1'22—dc23

                    2014021218

10 9 8 7 6 5 4 3 2 1

DESIGN BY DEBRA LONG HAMPTON

CONTENTS

INTRODUCTION

As I CONDUCT public presentations of true ghost experiences and describe how people in the South have encountered real ghosts in their everyday lives, I'm often asked where a person might go to see a ghost. My initial response is to suggest they stay home. Ghosts are all around us.

My second suggestion for people who want to visit a location where they are likely to encounter a ghost is to go to the hospital. The obvious reason is that a large number of people have died there. Many of those, especially in days of yore, experienced pain, isolation, desperation, dismemberment, dread, fear, or trauma. These, along with being separated from loved ones, are things known to create lasting ghosts.

Many abandoned hospitals, sanatoriums, and asylums are still standing in the South. Large buildings are costly to demolish. Other hospitals have been repurposed as hotels, apartment complexes, office buildings, and educational facilities. The structures are home to hundreds of ghosts, most of whom must wonder where all the patients went.

I need kindly to remind readers that no abandoned hospital should be visited without permission. Similarly, some haunted sites included in this collection are on private property where trespassers are not welcome. Many others, however, are open to the public. Often as not, haunted historical sites, include old hospitals, house museums.

Here in Dixie, a large number of mansions, civic buildings, and plantations were quickly converted to hospital use as battle after bloody battle during the War Between the States moved through our towns and cities. Standing structures near battlefields in even the deepest South saw use as both Confederate and Union hospitals, sometimes simultaneously. Many of those lovely antebellum buildings are standing proud after all those years and are preserved as historic sites.

Where no structures were available, emergency medical services for the wounded were provided in tents and outdoor fields adjacent to the battlefields, thus creating additional sites of hospital hauntings. Those who died were buried in unmarked graves, sometimes by the hundreds. And railroad cars and steamboats were converted to mobile hospitals.

The hellacious war also produced body piles and mass graves. I can think of no better source of ghosts. A hospital and surgery were part of our military bases and forts from the earliest days of our history. Quite a few are preserved as historic locations and even as national parks.

As I began to research hospital ghosts, I was taken aback by the large number of known hauntings. Almost every type of ghost and known ghostly manifestation occurs in hospitals and associated care facilities, and even at locations where hospitals are no longer standing. Sometimes, they're in the parking lot.

I discovered two ghosts haunting dental offices. I also located ghosts in a former veterinary hospital, a pharmacy, ambulances, and, yes, a first-aid kit and a stethoscope. The fatal crash of a medevac helicopter with the patient aboard created a unique ghost in South Carolina.

As I wrote the featured stories for each Southern state and described the numerous additional sightings, I found I didn't need to stretch to include a wide variety of locations. Home hospitals were common, including that of a man in Florida who built his mausoleum as a recovery room, a woman who attached her lover's amputated leg to her own in Mississippi, and a midwife who was tried for practicing witchcraft in Virginia. I discovered that the ghost of Zelda Fitzgerald, who died in a fire in a mental hospital, walks the streets of my hometown.

Ghosts in the South are of a particular flavor, no doubt. It is my belief that the dirt in the South is older and warmer than in other places. The culture of taking the time to listen to others is a trait of Southern hospitality. We don't rush through our stories. Ghosts, who have all the time of eternity, appreciate that fact.

And there really is something about moonlight in magnolias and old oaks draped in Spanish moss that is, if not magical, downright spooky. As spooky as an abandoned hospital at night.

I invite readers who have a further curiosity about ghosts to visit OurHauntedSouth.com at your leisure. There, you'll find a free instructional manual, "How to See a Ghost." The site is also home to true ghost encounters based on interviews I have conducted throughout the South. You'll also find accounts of hauntings from the other books of Southern ghosts I have written for John F. Blair, Publisher.

You don't have to believe in ghosts to drop by. Of the hundreds of people I have talked to who have experienced a ghost, about half had absolutely no belief in ghosts at the time of their first encounter. So it really doesn't matter if you believe in ghosts. They believe in you.

The ghost will see you now.

THE GHOST WILL SEE YOU NOW

ALABAMA

HAUNTED HANDS
OLD BLOUNT MEMORIAL HOSPITAL,
1000 LINCOLN AVENUE,
ONEONTA

A SURGEON'S HANDIWORK is exactly that—the result of a steady and practiced pair of hands.

After retiring from a profession that fit him like a glove, surgeon Dennis Anderson built birdhouses in the basement of his home in Birmingham. The birdhouses were carefully designed and precisely crafted. His signature was a perch made of a dowel rod placed sideways at the front of each house, held by a tiny end-frame he invented himself. In the beginning, each birdhouse had its own personality. A detail here and there that wasn't included in the others.

The retired doctor started out by selling them at the local crafts fair. But his heart wasn't in it. Now, he stacked the finished houses along two walls in the basement and left them there. His most recent work looked haphazard, even from a distance. Parts no longer lined up. Boards weren't cut straight. He could barely keep the paint in the right places.

His wife suggested he build something new. A boat, perhaps. He thought maybe she was right. Focusing on a new project might keep his hands from shaking. There might be time left to build something incredible. After all, time was all he had.

Dr. Anderson decided he would fashion a life-sized hand out of wood. It would be like a mannequin's hand, but different. He thought he would make a hand that could shake hands. Each finger would be intricately designed to open and close, to grip.

He never got the chance.

Years earlier, Dr. Anderson had retired from the practice of surgery in Birmingham when his hands began to shake at inopportune times. Nothing severe at the onset, but he knew better than to risk the health of patients by conducting surgery. He had enough money invested to live well enough in his final years.

At that time, Dr. Anderson took on part-time instructional and mentoring duties at Blount Memorial Hospital in Oneonta, thirty-five miles northeast of Birmingham. It was a small hospital, and the surgery was routine. He could handle it.

His knowledge of, and experience with, situations that might occur during surgery was vast. The residents and new surgeons looked up to him, asked his advice, and were always pleased to have Dr. Anderson assist in the operating room. He would sometimes open and close for them during a long or tedious surgery. At least, when his hands didn't shake, he did.

The palsy in his hands was a symptom of something worse to come. As a doctor, Dennis Anderson knew as much. He had tremor-onset Parkinson's disease. Drugs did little to help. In the beginning, the palsy, most noticeable in his hands, came and went. The doctor's hands would shake for a bit, then stop.

One day, however, he was unable to keep coffee from sloshing over the edges of his cup. The tremors would not stop. When he lifted the cup toward his mouth, he spilt hot coffee on himself. He left the hospital in Oneonta for good that day. Though he longed to go back, he was too embarrassed to return, too self-conscious to teach.

Upon his retirement, Dr. Anderson still had hours a day when his hands didn't shake. He went to work building birdhouses. His work was unsurpassed. Dennis Anderson was good at whatever he put a hand to. This was true for almost all of his life. But of late, it was true only most of the time. Then part of the time. And finally, for only a short time each day. And some days, not even that.

The morning he decided to craft a human hand wasn't a good one for Dr. Anderson.

Tremors shook his entire arm. He couldn't read his watch to see the time. It wouldn't stop moving long enough.

Dr. Anderson turned on his table saw. He had endured enough. He sliced his hand off at the wrist.

It hurt like a son of a gun, but the pain wasn't enough to stop him. Still standing, he sliced off his other hand on the spinning saw blade and went into shock. His watch hit the floor. Dr. Anderson no longer had time on his hands. He crumpled to his knees, fell forward, and bled out.

Later that day, his wife found him. Horrified, she understood. Dr. Andersen was taken to the funeral home after his body was checked by the county coroner. In consideration of the family, the coroner listed Dr. Anderson's death as an accident.

His wife didn't know what to do with his severed hands. If she let the mortician sew them back on, the skilled surgeon would surely be aghast at the stitching—at the fact that his veins were not sewn back together, nor the bones of his wrist repaired. And she couldn't display the body at visitation with his hands sitting atop his chest showing his wedding ring. The best she could do was to have her husband buried with his arms to his sides, half the casket open, and trust that the mortician had placed the hands in the casket somewhere out of view.

She had his wedding ring removed and displayed on his chest at the funeral.

Weeks afterward, Dr. Anderson's wife experienced a nightmare of seeing her husband lying with his hands behind his head. When he sat up to smile at her, the hands stayed on the pillow. Handless arms reached out to her. She woke in a sweat, panting, and whispered to her husband of all those years, "What do you want?"

And she heard him answer, "I want to go back to work."

Or maybe the question and answer were part of the dream. She didn't know what to think.

"Go right ahead, darling," she said. And for that part, she was as awake as you or I.

It is no secret that renovations and remodeling of long-existing structures may disturb ghosts. Some ghosts have been known to appear simply when furniture in its proper place when they died is later moved about.

When a new medical-arts building came into use in 1994, the original Blount Memorial Hospital in Oneonta was converted to offices. Workers reported more than one ghostly encounter while the former hospital was being remodeled. Unrelated to Dr. Anderson was the ghost of an unnamed child sitting under the window inside a former patient room. The youngster's shape was visible in dust particles as morning sunlight flooded the room. Seen simultaneously by two workers, the shape never moved, then disappeared as the light changed and the dust particles settled.

Another encounter came when an elderly man was installing smoke detectors in the new offices. While standing on a ladder, he felt hands run up his legs. He quickly surveyed his surroundings to see who was messing with him and discovered he was alone in the recently remodeled room. He left the ladder behind and hurriedly exited the room. He refused to return.

Current occupants of the offices note that incoming telephone calls are occasionally answered by someone who isn't there, who rapidly disconnects the call before it can be answered properly. One employee says her boyfriend has to phone three or four times in a row before the call goes through.

"Someone keeps hanging up on him," she says. "Maybe Dr. Andersen doesn't approve."

In winter, gloves left unattended will walk out of a room seemingly on their own. Some believe gloves left in the new offices at Blount Memorial Hospital are occupied by the severed hands of deceased surgeon Dennis Anderson. After all, his wife said he could come back if he wanted.

Should you be unable to find your gloves at Blount Memorial, rest assured they are in good hands. A bunch of baby birds in finely crafted houses mounted on poles and trees throughout the Birmingham area would agree. Mrs. Anderson donated her husband's remaining birdhouses, stacked in their basement, to the local Goodwill, which quickly sold every one.

THE GRATEFUL DEAD
OLD MOBILE GENERAL HOSPITAL,
900 BLOCK OF ST. ANTHONY STREET,
MOBILE

THE DAUGHTERS OF CHARITY managed and operated the old Mobile General Hospital for more than a hundred years. Victims of recurring yellow-fever epidemics in the 1850s in coastal Alabama were treated here. Also known as Mobile City Hospital, the massive Greek Revival structure was constructed beginning in 1830. That was the same year the brick wall was built around Church Street Cemetery, where a large number of yellow-fever victims from the hospital were interred.

Converted to office space in 1966, the hospital is now listed on the National Register of Historic Places. The building of stucco over brick features a long colonnaded front and portico supported by three-story Doric columns and is often visited by people interested in antebellum architecture of the Deep South.

There are other visitors. Some have never left the facility and, though dead for more than a century, continue to make Mobile City Hospital their home. These include a pair of young boys who have become the South's most prominent examples of the grateful dead.

Among known ghosts, the grateful dead provide perhaps the earliest examples of interactions between the living and the deceased. Lost souls of the departed express their thanks and provide rewards for favors performed by the living on their behalf.

At least two ghosts of the grateful dead currently inhabit Mobile City Hospital. One is Luke, who suffered a badly mangled leg when he

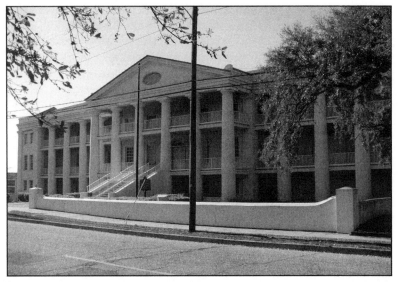

The Old Mobile City Hospital in Mobile, Alabama

was accidentally run over by a delivery wagon on the unpaved streets of old Mobile. Luke came to live at the hospital in the 1850s. Henry is his younger companion. Both are believed to be orphans of victims of yellow fever.

In describing the hospital in an April 27, 1857, article, the *Mobile Daily Register* noted, "The first floor is devoted to male patients, the second to females, and servants are accommodated in the spacious airy attic." The newspaper also made mention of the grounds and gardens at the rear and on each side of the hospital. The article failed to mention the morgue in the basement, though a large number of visitors at the time, and subsequently during the War Between the States, found their way there to retrieve the bodies of family members and loved ones.

During those years, Luke and Henry did what they could to help. Orphans under the care of the Daughters of Charity provided services to the hospital as a contribution toward the cost of their food, clothes, and board. Luke established himself as a bootblack for staff and visitors to the hospital. The polite and hardworking lad charged nothing to clean and shine shoes but gladly accepted tips from people who waited on the bench seats of the second-story entry to the hospital. Those who took a shine to Luke received a shine in return. One of the hospital surgeons stopped daily to have Luke polish his boots so he might place a coin in the hand of the industrious orphan.

At times when he wasn't handing shoe-shining materials to Luke, Henry happily guided visitors to the various rooms of the hospital. Then he quickly returned to assist his older companion, who sometimes fell when he moved too rapidly on his bad leg. Henry carried Luke's box when the bootblack found it necessary to hobble up or down the hospital stairs, assuring that neither orphan was late for lunch or supper.

When a coin was proffered for services, the two orphans always said thank you.

Both Luke and Henry donated every cent and half-cent they received to the Daughters of Charity. No one knows the outcomes of their lives. No one knows how long they lived or where they died. No one can quite remember when the bootblack was no longer there. But it has been noted that a smiling old man with a bad leg polished shoes in the hospital lobby in the 1920s. At about that time, an aged Confederate veteran visiting the hospital tipped him a twenty-dollar gold piece for polishing his boots. The hunched-over bootblack said thank you.

What is known for certain is that both boys have chosen to stay in the hospital beyond their deaths, fixed in place at the time of their youthful service to others. To this day, the faces of children are seen in the upper windows of the former Mobile City Hospital late at night. And more importantly, their voices are still heard.

To this day, visitors to the historic building report that when a coin is dropped on the lobby floor, they hear the voice of a young boy saying thank you. Whether it is Henry or Luke, no one is sure. But surely, it is the voice of the grateful dead.

While both boys knew every corner of the structure—from the

morgue in the basement to the treatment and recovery rooms to the kitchen to the attic cubbyholes—the ghosts of Luke and Henry seem to have mastered the elevator that was later installed. Those who work in the offices of the remodeled building note that the elevator door sometimes opens when approached before the button can be pushed. People in Mobile who receive this preferential treatment know it is common courtesy—a custom not yet expired in the South—to say thank you to the empty elevator. Some even say, "Thank you, Henry," or "Thank you, Luke."

At the old Mobile General Hospital, gratitude is a door that swings both ways. Between the living and the dead.

OLD BONES, NEW BONES

JEMISON CENTER,
WEST OF THE AIRPORT OFF FIFTH STREET,
NORTHPORT

IN THE 1930s, Mavis Denny provided important services to residents of the Jemison Center, a state-run mental hospital for African-Americans in Northport, Alabama. Mavis slept in the nurses' quarters behind the main building, where she worked seven days a week as a cook. She also divined the future for individuals by reading bones. Not their bones, of course.

Mavis kept her eclectic mix of divining bones in a wooden cigar box in her room. Divining bones were a mix of old and new bones, but always small bones. Some were no larger than the tip of a finger or a little toe.

Her client one night was a nurse who worked and lived at the Jemison Center.

They sat on the floor. Like so many, Miss Stevens was worried about her love life. She rattled the box of bones and dumped the contents between her and Mavis. Once the bones tumbled into place, Mavis studied the map.

Nothing was there. She scratched her head.

"Do it again," she said. "And this time, hold my hand."

Miss Stevens complied.

Still nothing. The bones were silent.

"We'll try again tomorrow," Mavis assured her disappointed client.

Mavis needed a new bone to bring life to her divinations. She'd pull one out and put one in. She always kept the oldest.

Rabbit bones were the best for showing a person's course through the world, represented by a few odd squirrel bones. A gopher bone was always good for helping find lost items. Small bones of cats or possums showed the way through the darkness that surrounds all of us. Bones from a crow defined that darkness. These were the old bones, since evils in life rarely changed. The fixes people found themselves in were about the same from one decade to the next.

Mavis defined the individual darkness for a client. She would read where and when evil would drop its veil in their lives, and advise them how to protect themselves, how to have the evil fall to the side, and how best to proceed to find brightness and joy.

She regularly required a new bone to keep her divining fresh. Rarely, though, had Mavis drawn a complete blank when reading bones. More than a fresh bone from a burrowing mole or a felled sparrow was called for. She needed the real thing this time. Shiny and white and little. A boiled bone that would tumble.

When her client was gone, Mavis slipped away from the nurses' quarters and made her way in darkness to the back door of the Jemison Center. She found a heavy knife with a sharp blade in the kitchen and took it with her to the morgue. Sorely disappointed to discover that none of the 250 or so patients had died that week, she hid the knife in her clothes and briefly returned to her quarters to retrieve a sewing kit she kept in the drawer of her bedside table.

The nurse on duty in the women's ward noticed Mavis when she looked up from her magazine and said hello.

"Awfully late to be here tonight," the nurse said. "It's almost midnight."

The night nurse, a regular client of Mavis Denny's readings, worried that something as yet unforetold was about to be revealed to her, something so devastating the fortune teller could wait no longer to bring her the news.

"Late for some, early for others," Mavis said, smiling. Midnight was a perfect time to snatch a toe. The hour was downright magical. "I need to see someone."

The nurse relaxed, then nodded, relieved that Mavis was there to see someone else. Anyone else.

Mavis walked the hallway to the rooms at the far end. She slipped inside a room where the most demented were housed, heavily sedated and strapped into their beds. She turned on the lights and found a foot with handsome, long toes. She cut off the end bone of a little toe. The patient stirred inside her thick leather straps without waking. Mavis sewed her up without blinking.

In the kitchen, she placed a pot of water on one of the burners. The bone had to be boiled, of course.

The next night, Mavis told Miss Stevens it was time to try another reading. Once in position, the nurse scattered the cigar box of small bones between them on the floor. This time, it was all there. One little white bone stood out among the rest. Old bones and new bones together told a story she was eager to share.

"Your life is about to turn in new ways," Mavis said. "You will be leaving here soon. Very soon. A man you already know will come for you."

Mavis Denny died long before the mental institution closed. Through the 1960s, patients, families, and visitors complained of the deterioration of the facility since its construction in the 1920s. Patients fared no better than the buildings. In 1970, a journalist for the *Tuscaloosa News* reported on what many considered inhumane conditions at the Jemison Center. "One tiny shower closet served 131 male patients," he wrote. "The 75 women patients also had but one shower." The article noted that urine saturated the aging oak floors, that many occupied beds lacked linens, and that some patients slept on the floors. "Most patients at Jemison were highly tranquilized," the reporter added. "All appeared to lack any semblance of treatment."

The Jemison Center closed within the next few years and was completely abandoned.

When claims surfaced that the buildings were haunted, the deteriorating and empty facility quickly became a hangout for local high-school students and college students from nearby Tuscaloosa. The buildings today, though still standing, are in ruin. Visiting the Jemison Center without permission is not allowed. Northport police visit the grounds frequently to check for and detain trespassers.

Still, curiosity seekers make their way to the Jemison Center, where they find that the buildings are not always as empty as they seem. Nearly everyone reports a feeling of being watched from the corners of rooms when no one else is there. Reports of furniture being moved to block return passage along hallways are common, as are reports of frigid spots when the temperature is otherwise warm.

Sensing a ghost is not the scariest thing that has happened to visitors to the Jemison Center. Not by far.

On a sunny afternoon in the spring of 2002, two female students from the University of Alabama in Tuscaloosa carried a Ouija board, a candle, and a folding card table into the main building of the Jemison Center. They carefully made their way through the general destruction and graffiti-covered walls to the second floor.

Sunlight streamed through the broken windows. Except for occasional cold spots, the rooms were cozy and warm, even those cluttered with debris. They stopped when they came upon a patient room with two old chairs and a dilapidated bed. They set up the table, slapped the dust and dirt from the chairs as best they could, and positioned the chairs and themselves on opposite sides of the folding table.

"I guess we wanted to be witches," Terri Bonham said. "We'd both watched the movie *Practical Magic* about a hundred times, and we'd heard that the old hospital was supposed to be inhabited by spirits of the dead. I know it sounds stupid, but Marcia and I wanted to see if we could get someone from the other side to light the candle for us."

Terri and Marcia set up the Ouija board and placed the unlit candle on the table.

"I'd heard somewhere never to use a Ouija board to contact ghosts," Terri said. "Because the process invites a spirit to intervene on your behalf, it's considered dangerous. When you invite a spirit to join you, it may never leave. All that just made it more fun, we thought."

Once everything was arranged, two hands rested on the windowed planchette of the board.

"Is anyone here?" Terri asked out loud.

The plastic planchette moved under their fingers to reveal the answer: Yes.

"I got scared at that point," Terri confessed. "But Marcia wanted to know the spirit's name."

The planchette moved across the surface, spelling out *M-A-V-I-S* on the board. The two girls were instantly chilled. Terri said it felt like an ice cube had moved up her spine. And when the spirit finished her name, both girls felt something, or someone, pull their toes.

"That was it for both of us. We weren't waiting around for the candle to light on its own."

The two college girls scrambled off the old chairs. Pushing each other out of the way, tripping over upturned furniture and chunks of plaster on the floor, Terri and Marcia raced from the room, down the cluttered stairs, and out of the building. Terri had snatched up the Oujia board, gladly leaving behind the card table, the planchette, and the unlit candle.

The girls discovered that each of them had stubbed their toes on their haphazard dash to safety. Terri, in fact, had lost a shoe. Her little toe was cut and bleeding. But it was there. She limped to the car, insisting that something had pulled off her shoe while they were still at the Oujia board.

"We later learned that our Mavis might be Mavis Denny needing new bones," Terri said. "It was the first time I'd heard the story of the bones lady who told fortunes at the Jemison Center. And I surely believe it's true because that's not all that happened."

For the rest of the spring semester, while the cut on Terri's toe healed, the college roommates would feel someone pulling their toes when they were asleep in the dorm.

"I mean a hard pull, not just a little tug," Terri insisted. "It would wake us up and, when it did, it was always midnight or a minute after."

The girls, it seemed, had been followed home by a former resident of the Jemison Center.

During finals, Terri and Marcia decided to put an end to it. They returned to the abandoned hospital in Northport. This time, they brought along two boys.

"I wasn't going back in there," Terri explained. "And I told them if they found my shoe, to leave it there. I didn't want it back."

The boys, with Marcia as a guide, carried the Ouija board back to the room on the second floor. The folding table was still in place. Terri's shoe was under the table. A spider had built its web across the laces, which were untied.

One of the boys opened the Ouija board and positioned it on the card table. Marcia found the planchette and candle on the floor. She put the planchette on the table and set the candle upright next to the board.

As one might give commands to an obedient dog, Marcia said three times aloud for Mavis to stay. She and the boys then left the room.

Neither girl has since been troubled by midnight toe tugs. And neither has visited the Jemison Center again. Terri advises against going there.

"Jemison Center's dead fortune teller may or may not live in that room," she said. "But wherever she is, I know one thing. Mavis Denny needs new bones."

OTHER ALABAMA SIGHTINGS

ANNISTON

The Blue Ridge Mountains are said to end just outside Anniston, Alabama. But Stringfellow Memorial Hospital in Anniston is home to two haunts that never end. Susie Parker Stringfellow, who willed the land for the hospital upon her death in 1920, loved to play the organ. She still does. Her phantom music routinely emanates from the hospital chapel when no one is sitting at the organ.

A fifty-eight-year-old resident of Anniston died at Stringfellow Memorial Hospital in mid-December 1989, shortly after being diagnosed with cancer. An article in the *Anniston Star* detailed his death the day after it occurred, quoting a family friend as saying the deceased had "wanted to call the shots." That's exactly what he did. The patient brought a gun to the hospital and committed suicide by shooting himself in the head. The gunshot dislodged portions of his face. The haunting created by that violent trauma has resulted in the occasional sighting of a headless ghost in the Stringfellow Memorial hallways. Others have observed the apparition of an eyeball rolling across the floor and out the door of the room in which the patient took his life. The eyeball always appears in December and ceases on the twenty-fifth. Many suspect the patient simply wants to see one more Christmas.

AUBURN

Auburn University Chapel, built in 1851 as a Presbyterian church, subsequently served as a Confederate hospital. The chapel is haunted by an impatient Brit, Sydney Grimlett, who served in the war as a Confederate soldier. Grimlett had his leg amputated at the makeshift hospital following a shrapnel injury from a Union cannonball in 1864. Rumors that he died during amputation are false. Grimlett survived for years after the war and often attended services at the Presbyterian church, where he was intent on getting a leg up on any Sunday pulpit-pounding he believed carried on too long.

Grimlett, it seems, believed that anything that can be done right can also be done expeditiously. The old soldier rapidly tapped his wooden leg on the floor when the sermon didn't end quickly enough. And he kept on tapping, louder and louder from a back pew, until the preaching concluded. For decades, parishioners took delight in advising new preachers that the tapping, once it began, would not end until they stopped talking. Sunday lunches were always on time.

Sold to the university in 1921, the church for years housed the Auburn Players Theater, where Grimlett, still present though long dead, was heard to tap his wooden leg from one of the seats in the auditorium in an effort to end lengthy rehearsals. It was also discovered that Grimlett enjoyed a good show. As long as the actors ended on time, his wooden leg hit the floor over and over in rapid succession during the applause at the end of each public performance.

After undergoing significant renovation, the historic building, listed on the National Register of Historic Places, became a church again in 1976 and now serves as the interdenominational Auburn University Chapel.

CITRONELLE

It is a common occurrence among hauntings that some people continue their life's work after they're dead. Perhaps this is from habit, and the ghosts don't know what else they might do. In other examples, the ghosts appear totally dedicated to a task.

Such is the haunting on the streets of Citronelle, a small town in extreme southeast Alabama. A body wagon draws slowly down the street to stop in front of homes where a person is dying. It is never seen. The rhythmic fall of horse hooves and the creaking of wooden wheels are the first indications the ghost is approaching. When the ghost wagon stops, a male voice announces, "Here for your dead, Captain."

The horse and wagon, along with the snap of the reins in the driver's hands, are also heard passing along Citronelle's three-mile gas-lit walking trail. The wagon's destination is unknown, although locals speculate the driver is carrying the dead to a better place.

CULLMAN

A ghost named Homer, usually seen as an elderly man in a hospital gown, is well known to the former staff of the old Woodland Hospital in Cullman, Alabama. Recently renovated, the facility currently serves as the Sanctuary of the Woods, a psychiatric hospital specializing in geriatric care. According to recent reports, Homer still shows up on an unoccupied gurney whenever he feels like it. Staffers believe Homer is waiting to be taken somewhere. This may be an example of a ghost who is lost and seeking to find his way to the other side. In Homer's case, he's waiting for a ride.

GADSDEN

There are many places children are told not to go for their own safety. But as all parents know, children sometimes go where they aren't supposed to. And ghosts, as we learn through experience, do pretty much what people do. Or at least they try to.

Mountain View Hospital is situated above the Coosa River in Gadsden, Alabama. The ghost of a child is situated there as well. He is seen from inside the rooms, sitting out on the fire escape. One suspects he's been told not to. Perhaps that's why he's always smiling.

LESTER

The abandoned D. E. Jackson Memorial Hospital in Lester, Alabama, is the current venue for an annual haunted house tour for charity. But one guest from the other side is known to haunt the parking lot of the facility year-round.

Locally known as "the Bride of Lesterstein," the walking apparition of a woman in a blood-covered wedding gown crisscrosses the parking area outside the former emergency room. The ghost bride lifts her bloody veil to peer into the front and rear seats of cars parked near the closed facility at night. When she doesn't find what she is seeking, the Bride of Lesterstein walks away and then disappears.

The recurring ghastly visage is that of an area bride who was fatally injured in a car wreck on the way to her wedding. She died while being transferred from the ambulance to the emergency room at Jackson Memorial. More importantly, perhaps, the bloodied young lady died before her soon-to-be husband arrived at the hospital, and there's something she longs to tell him.

Locals believe the wedding ghost will go away once she finds who she is looking for and utters the words, "I do." Others suggest she is likely to hang on for the honeymoon.

MONTEVALLO

When darkness falls at the University of Montevallo, a security detail comprised of one ghost appears outside Reynolds Hall.

Constructed in 1851, Reynolds Hall served as a Confederate hospital late in the War Between the States. It now provides space for Theater Department classes and rehearsals. An officer and a gentleman to the end and beyond, the ghost of Captain Henry Clay Reynolds, for whom the building is named, escorts university students to their dormitories at night. A nocturnal apparition, the gallant captain lingers two steps behind walking students until they safely reach their destinations.

MOUNT VERNON

Searcy Mental Hospital, a state psychiatric treatment and housing facility for African-Americans, was established in 1902 on the grounds of the former Mount Vernon Arsenal. A five-story guard tower makes the location easily identifiable today—as does the face of a former patient seen in one of the windows.

Searcy was desegregated in 1969. Listed on the National Register of Historic Places, the facility was closed in 2012. Ghost faces seen in the windows of closed buildings are common phenomena of the South. At

Searcy in particular, the former patient's visage seems to be embedded in the glass. It can be seen from outside the building only when viewed from a particular angle and when the light is just right.

One theory is that the face of the woman is attached to the object—that is, trapped inside the pane of glass. Rather than inhabiting the room on the other side of the window, the ghost is a physical imprint in the glass itself. The face, like a handprint in concrete, is thus an artifact. Some researchers believe that, should the window be broken, the ghost face will become fragments impossible to reconstruct. It will be gone.

Other who aren't so sure suggest the face would appear in another window were the current one to be broken, or would continue to be seen whether glass is there or not.

When you see the face of the ghost, witnesses insist, the ghost sees you.

SELMA

Two blocks from the Alabama River in Selma is the three-story Vaughan-Smitherton Museum. Constructed in 1847, it was formerly the old Vaughan Memorial Hospital, which closed in 1969.

The carefully maintained grounds are not the only thing of beauty here. So is the voice of a nurse who cared for a large number of Confederate soldiers who suffered injuries at the Battle of Selma on April 2, 1865, one week prior to General Robert E. Lee's surrender at Appomattox. The young nurse celebrated the cooling rains in Selma by singing as she walked the hospital hallways. Her refreshing moments of joy linger today. The nurse's lilting voice can be heard in the gardens and along the corridor of the third-floor of the museum whenever it rains.

TUSCALOOSA

One of several historic buildings on the ever-expanding University of Alabama campus, the columned Bryce Hospital is the state's oldest inpatient psychiatric facility. The hospital is currently undergoing renovation for educational use.

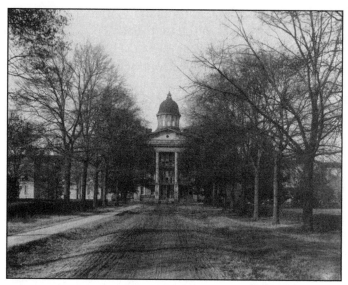

Bryce Hospital for the Insane, circa 1907

The first recorded burials at Bryce date to 1861. It is estimated that thousands of graves on the grounds remain unmarked. The ghost of a man who died at Bryce Hospital and was buried nearby wanders in seemingly aimless circles upon the land surrounding the building. Clad in rags, the ghost carries a tin cup and quietly offers those who are dead and buried a drink of water. When approached by the living, he disappears into the ground.

ARKANSAS

TO HAVE A BODY
OLD BAPTIST MEMORIAL HOSPITAL,
1 PERSHING CIRCLE,
NORTH LITTLE ROCK

WHILE STAN GILBERT WAS UNDERGOING a routine gallbladder removal at Baptist Memorial Hospital in North Little Rock, his monitor sounded a warning. Stan was fifty-eight.

"Heart!" the anesthesiologist said, alerting the surgery team. He adjusted the amount of anesthesia and circled behind the top of Stan's head.

The surgeon conducting the open cholecystectomy paused. He was concerned he might lose any patient during surgery, but surely not during a gallbladder procedure.

A nurse in surgical cap, mask, gloves, and gown stepped forward and prepared to administer a two-hand heart massage. She placed one hand over the other one on the patient's chest.

It wasn't needed. Stan's heartbeat returned on its own, and the surgery continued.

His first night home from the hospital, Stan woke in the middle of the night when his pain meds wore off. He needed to use the bathroom. And take another pill.

Stan hated the pills. Whenever he took one, the smell of the hospital returned. It was a smell he could taste on his tongue and the roof of his mouth. But he needed help with the abdominal pain if he was going to sleep, which was about the only thing he'd done since coming home.

On his way to the bathroom, Stan walked into a wall that shouldn't have been there. He knocked a painting down that almost hit his feet when it slid to the floor.

This isn't good, he thought. He was out of it. Nothing felt right.

As the bottom of the framed painting hit the carpet, his wife sat up in bed.

Stan stared at the painting. It was of a clown. And it was rather badly done. Nothing felt right because nothing was right.

"Darling, is that you?" his wife asked, and turned on the lamp at her bedside table. Her heart leapt. She knew he would return to her. At least once. Soul mates always say goodbye before they move on.

Stan turned to look at his wife. It was a woman he'd never seen before. She had blond hair and was far too young to be married to him.

He was suddenly dizzy. Then his legs faltered. Stan dropped to the bedroom carpet, which was the wrong color to begin with, and stared at what looked like a red banana. It was the clown's mouth. He prayed there would be no clowns in heaven. His eyes wide open, Stan soon saw nothing.

In a different house in Little Rock, Barbara Gilbert told paramedics that he was like that when she woke up. Cold. Blue. Not breathing. "It must have been his heart," she said. She was still holding her husband's hand. She kissed his cold fingers. Her tears wouldn't end.

The paramedics placed his body on the ambulance gurney as Stan's niece arrived to comfort Barbara. Secretly, Barbara blamed the medications. All else had gone well for Stan, according to the hospital.

As with all large hospitals, more than one life hung in the balance at Baptist Memorial the moment Stan's heart went on the blink during gallbladder surgery. A young father named Michael Alquist had been ushered into an adjoining operating room for emergency surgery after being backed over by a large truck at the loading dock where he worked. His legs were crushed and his pelvis badly damaged. He'd lost a lot of blood.

Michael was in shock. Immediate surgery was required to keep him alive. But surgery and shock do not mix well. The goal of saving the young father's life proved out of reach of the medical staff. He died of his injuries before repairs could be made.

"Your father was here last night," Mrs. Alquist told her daughter the morning of his burial. "I saw him in the room. He took the painting I did in high school off the wall and set it on the floor. Then he went away."

Trying not to cry, the daughter smiled as best she could manage and said nothing.

"Only he was older," Mrs. Alquist said. "He had white hair and had gained a lot of weight."

She carried the painting to the funeral home that day and propped it against the casket. She was comforted to know that Michael could walk on the other side, even though his legs had been crushed at the end of his life. She didn't care that his hair had turned white on the other side.

Stan Gilbert was buried a few days later. Headstones for Stan and Michael were placed on the appropriate graves, identifying the resting places of the bodies.

Bodies are one thing. Spirits are another.

Many ghosts are trapped in one place. But spirits who wander must find a means. Some accomplish this by attaching themselves to an object. When the object is moved, the ghost comes along.

Others are content to visit the living only in dreams. Michael died after his legs and pelvis were crushed by a delivery truck. He died before his injuries could be repaired. He didn't want his wife to see his mangled body. Michael feared such a visit would be horrible for her.

As a ghost, then, he was pretty much limited to showing up as a voice and nothing more. Or as an empty weight by her side in bed. That wasn't enough for Michael. So when the opportunity arose, he became a body sharer.

Michael treated Stan like a vacation rental. The door was left unattended when Stan's heart stopped beating during surgery to removal his gallbladder. Michael, only moments deceased, slipped inside. He moved in for the weekend and pretty much had the run of the place. At least while Stan was sleeping.

When Stan woke up, Michael ducked behind a chair, darted behind the curtains, or dove under the bed. The ghost hid in the corners of his temporary abode, but he was always there.

Michael used Stan to visit his wife in his own home. Stan woke up unexpectedly. He woke at the wrong time and in the wrong place. Although Michael's wife saw only the ghost image of his living body, Stan saw her. The shock of having been transported to another place, a place he'd never seen before, was too much for his weakened heart to overcome.

As Stan died staring at the painting of a clown, his body returned without Michael to where it had always been.

And Michael's spirit returned to the location of his own death. He moved from room to room at the old hospital for the next several years, looking for a body to briefly borrow and occasionally finding one.

The old Baptist Memorial Hospital was recently demolished. It is not considered a safe place to visit. Unless, that is, you're looking to bring someone home with you and to go new places the next time you fall asleep.

THE TOWEL SCREAMER
BATHHOUSE ROW AND THE GRAND PROMENADE, HOT SPRINGS

SOME GHOSTS ARE HEARD. Some ghosts are seen. At Hot Springs National Park, a well-known ghost is never seen without being heard. And is never heard without being seen.

Her name is Antonia Camello. She and her husband motored south from Chicago to take the restorative cure in the thermal baths at Hot Springs. They drove carefully, hugging the rising and falling curves through the forested Ozark and Ouachita mountains. Although the mountains were small, the forest seemed primeval. Dogwoods bloomed in the shade of taller trees. Running streams appeared around every turn.

Paul said it all started with the Indians.

"Indians knew what was good for you," he informed his wife. "They never went to the doctor."

"Medicine man," Antonia said.

"What?"

"They had a medicine man."

"Hocus-pocus," her husband scoffed. "They didn't go to no medicine man. They went to the springs. Indians didn't have arthritis, polio, or cancer. What they had was hot springs."

"Think hot water's a cure for stupidity?" Antonia asked.

"If it's good enough for the president of the United States, it's good enough for me. FDR's no dunce."

In an 1818 treaty, the Quapaw Indians ceded the interior Arkansas highlands, including the hot springs, to the United States. Arkansas became a territory soon afterward. The territorial legislature requested that

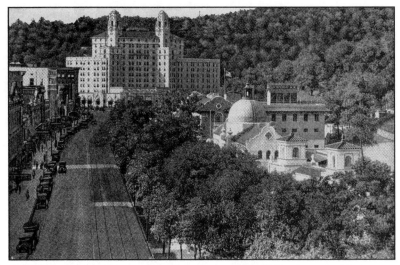

Central Avenue in Hot Springs, Arkansas, looking north. Bathhouse Row, circa 1924, is on the right.

the springs and adjoining mountains be set aside as a federal reserve. The request was eventually granted. Established in 1832, the reserve was named Hot Springs National Park in 1921.

A million gallons a day of naturally heated water, rich in mineral content, flow from springs on the western slope of Hot Springs Mountain in the city's historic downtown. The water percolates deep in the earth's crust until it becomes overheated. It then rushes to the surface to emerge at a temperature of 143 degrees. A channel of the heated spring water, known as Hot Springs Creek, runs underground from an area near Park Avenue to the famed Bathhouse Row, which consists of eight turn-of-the-twentieth-century historic spa buildings fronted by a formal promenade, all managed by the National Park Service. Fordyce Bathhouse serves as the park's visitor center.

When Antonia and her husband arrived in the spring of 1936, Hot Springs was noted for its gangsters and gambling. And the luxurious

Fordyce was at peak operation. Financed by Samuel Fordyce as a standing testament to the healing waters to which he believed he owed his own life, the bathhouse was the most elaborate of the spa structures on Bathhouse Row. The Fordyce, of a decidedly Mediterranean Renaissance Revival design, opened in 1915. It offered all the spa treatments available in the other bathhouses and had a bowling alley and a billiards room thrown in for good measure. It also boasted a gymnasium and a roof garden for fresh air and sunbathing. Stately rooms were set aside for conversation and reading.

Of course, the main thing was the therapeutic baths. A hot bath was good for what ailed you. Add a massage and you had the very definition of physical therapy. And indeed, people trusted bathhouses to provide relief for a variety of ailments.

Often called "hot-water hospitals," bathhouses proffered a cure for just about everything through hydrotherapy. It didn't hurt that the therapy was for the most part enjoyable. Consumers were additionally romanced with the notion that the mineral content of spring water was magically curative.

Various spas across America developed special hydrotherapy treatments for heart disease and circulatory disorders, rheumatic conditions, nervous disorders, metabolic diseases, obesity, digestive ailments, and skin diseases, including acne and psoriasis. Hot Springs was no exception. Rumors circulated that, if you got there soon enough, bathing in and drinking the mineral-rich hot water would cure syphilis.

People were being lured to springs of bubbling hot mineral water long before there was written history. Archaeological digs at the site of natural hot springs in France and the Czech Republic have uncovered sufficient Bronze Age artifacts to conclude that gatherings at, and pilgrimages to, the thermal waters were routine.

Paul Camello's 1935 Hudson Terraplane was only one in a long line of automobiles to make its way along the Arkansas mountain roads to find the hot baths at the end its journey. And maybe some gambling. Two fellows he knew in Chicago had horses running that weekend at Oaklawn

Park, the racetrack just down the road from Bathhouse Row.

He and Antonia stayed at the Arlington Hotel, located at the corner of Central Avenue and Fountain Street. It's where Al Capone stayed when he was in Hot Springs.

"Don't say nothing about that to nobody," Paul instructed his wife. "He might be there while we are, and he doesn't like being talked about."

"Don't worry. I won't say anything to Al Capone." Antonia rolled down the window, then added, "Unless he asks me to dance."

Maybe she shouldn't have been so flip about old Scarface. Maybe Paul had his reasons for worrying.

Nobody asked Antonia to dance. They didn't get the chance. She slept in on Saturday and stayed in her room the rest of the day, ordering room service for lunch. Then she worked on her nails. Paul was supposed to return from the track in time for their therapy reservations at the Fordyce. He was drunk by the time he showed up.

"Two hundred bucks, can you believe it? I made us two hundred bucks." Paul felt like a king. He'd nailed the winner in the Arkansas Derby. "I'm naming our first kid Holl." Holl Image was the name of the horse Paul had wagered on to finish first in the feature race.

"That's nice, honey. Hurry up or we'll miss our baths."

"Ain't you hungry or something? Let's get a drink."

"You've had enough," she said. Antonia grabbed his hand and pulled him down the hall.

At the Fordyce, they undressed in separate rooms and were submerged in deep, heated water. Attendants washed their bodies with sponges. Then they were rubbed down on cooling tables and left to linger in what for Antonia was a state of serene bliss.

When she was sufficiently serene. Antonia wrapped a towel around herself and set off to find her husband. As drunk as he was, he'd probably fallen asleep. It was dark outside now. She was hungry.

Before she could find him, however, he found her. Paul barreled naked and wet down the Fordyce hallway, his feet slipping on the marble floor. One side of his face was red and swollen.

"They tried to kill me," he said. Paul grabbed her by the shoulders and pushed her out of the way. "Get out of here. They tried to drown me." Paul was past her now, running naked back to the room where he'd left his clothes in a locker. His gun was there. He'd rip the door off the locker if he had to.

He turned a corner. She heard the shots. Paul hadn't made it to the locker. Whoever was trying to kill him had gone the back way and cut him off.

It took a moment. She took two steps, following his wet tracks. Then she stopped.

Two men in suits splashed with water appeared at the end of the hall. One of them was smiling. They each held a hand inside their jackets.

Antonia backed up. Wearing only a towel, she turned and ran.

A shot rang out. It missed.

As she managed her barefoot way around a corner, she screamed. She found an exit at the back of the Fordyce and rushed into the night, still screaming, towel flapping. There was a trail behind the Fordyce for strolls. It was being covered in bricks. Antonia ran to her left.

Her towel fell. She stopped to pick it up and screamed again when she saw the two men jogging after her. Antonia made it to the last bathhouse and a little beyond, where the walking path turned uphill. There, she was shot by one of the Chicago gangsters who had killed her husband. She stumbled, wrapping the towel more tightly around her.

Another shot from a pistol and she dropped. Antonia stopped screaming.

"Had to be done. She saw us," one of the men said to the other.

The dampened duo slowed to catch their breath and walked by the lady in the towel on their way to the Arlington. Inside the crowded bar, one of them nodded to Capone, letting him know the job was over.

Casual visitors to Hot Springs today are likely to confuse the Magnolia Walkway in front of Bathhouse Row with the Grand Promenade, which is a brick walkway behind the architecturally diverse bathhouses. The half-mile promenade runs roughly parallel to Central Avenue and

Bathhouse Row, offering views of historic downtown, Arlington Lawn, the hot springs cascade, and the quartz veins in the sandstone and tufa cliffs. The promenade was named a National Recreation Trail in 1982.

Those near the entrance to the promenade during evening hours are likely to see a towel-clad ghost who runs screaming from the Fordyce Bathhouse on to the promenade and continues for approximately a quarter-mile before disappearing. The ghost is described as having curly blond hair and being of short stature with a curvaceous torso.

Tourists on the front walkway report hearing a woman scream at night and seeing flashes of a white towel moving between the bathhouses. Although Al Capone is not known to have killed anyone during his numerous vacations to Hot Springs, someone did. And Antonia is still screaming about it.

Some are likely to note that the most impressive space in the Fordyce is the third-floor assembly room, which has a ceiling of segmented, arched vaults with elaborate stained-glass skylights. Others say it's the towel-dressed woman running out the back door.

GRAVE HOSPITALITY
CRESCENT HOTEL,
25 PROSPECT AVENUE,
EUREKA SPRINGS

A MOUNTAINTOP RESORT AND SPA, the Crescent Hotel in Eureka Springs, Arkansas, was built in 1886. Recently named one of America's "Dozen Distinctive Destinations" by the National Trust for Historic Preservation, the hotel formerly served as a last-chance hospital opened by Norman G. Baker in 1937. A flamboyant millionaire inventor and radio personality, Baker styled himself a doctor, although he had absolutely no medical training.

Lack of knowledge of the causes and treatment of diseases didn't stop Baker, a former vaudeville magician, from claiming he had discovered a cure for cancer. Run out of Iowa for practicing medicine without a license, he relocated his cancer treatment to the Crescent Hotel, which had fallen on hard times during the Depression. He renamed the stone edifice the Baker Cancer Hospital and advertised his fictional cure.

The quack's cure for cancer primarily consisted of drinking water from the area's natural springs. It also included injections of glycerin. Critically ill patients were offered an exclusive elixir of tea brewed from watermelon seeds and clover, heavily laced with alcohol.

Because Baker used the mail for sending out brochures full of empty promises and fictional testimonials, he faced federal charges of fraud and was arrested in 1940 as a medical charlatan. An investigator estimated that Baker had defrauded cancer patients out of $4 million and that, instead of helping any of them, he had hastened their deaths.

His hospital was shut down. Not soon enough, however. Under Baker's care, a large number of desperately ill patients died, many of whom were buried in the basement of the so-called hospital.

Deviously deceitful and dishonest, the phony doctor nonetheless was in possession of certain charms, one of which was his manner of dress. Baker was described by his biographers as being handsome, with wavy white hair and hypnotic eyes. He was known for his trademark purple suits, shirts, and ties. He also drove a purple car. Baker is said to have been able to talk anyone into believing anything, not unlike some radio personalities today.

It is impossible to calculate the number of his victims. A woman named Theodora was one. Dying of cancer, she came under Baker's counterfeit care in 1938 with her husband of many years. The two shared a room on the fourth floor, where Theodora occupied a hospital bed. Her husband, Lenny, slept in a twin bed next to hers.

"I just want to sleep in a clean bed," she told her husband. "That's really all I want."

Theodora had no appetite for food or entertainment. Her cancer had spread throughout her body. The disease erupted in skin lesions. She was covered in sores. Worse, her vital organs and glands were quickly succumbing to the errant cells.

Lenny hoped for comfort for his wife, believing that Baker's treatment might alleviate her suffering, as well as potentially reverse the cancer's progress. Of course, the doses of Baker's phony cure accomplished neither.

The best that Lenny could manage was to arrive with his own treatment. He was, after all, a highly trained medical doctor of many years' experience. He carried two tins and a glass vial in his pockets at all times. The first tin held Anacin tablets for pain. The second held a supply of a newly developed sleep aid, hydrocodone. The vial contained a lethal amount of morphine.

As Baker's treatment proved ineffective for Theodora, Lenny found he was nearly out of hydrocodone. He gave his wife the last of it. She moaned with every shallow breath.

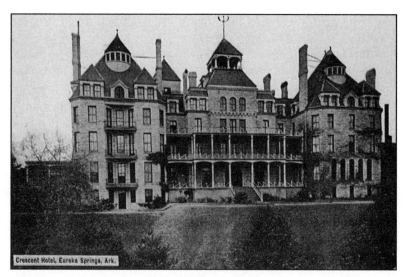

Crescent Hotel in Eureka Springs, Arkansas, circa 1886

Theodora thrashed against the pain in her arms, legs, and chest as he lifted her from the hospital bed and placed her emaciated body in a leather chair. Lenny pulled the untouched linens from his bed and used them to replace hers. He rested his wife on clean sheets and tried to soothe her discomfort and distress. It was impossible.

As she writhed in torment, he laid his body on top of hers to hold her still. Lenny held his wife's mouth open with one hand and fed her the lethal dose of morphine. Soon, she was calm. Theodora smiled in her narcotic trance, as if to say thank you. He prayed she was seeing heaven as she died.

Lenny stretched out beside his wife on the hospital bed. He lifted her hand time and time again to press his lips against her cold fingers. He shed the tears of angels. Later, Lenny sealed her eyes shut with two trembling, lingering kisses.

The official cause of death, certified in writing by the coroner, was malignant tumors of the lungs, complicated by additional cancerous tumors and lesions. But that wasn't true. Cancer had taken her life, for sure, but morphine had killed her. Her true cause of death, however, was love.

If people asked, Lenny was tempted to blame her death on Baker's "cure." But blame had nothing to do with Baker this time. Blame was something to be settled between Lenny and God.

Today, Baker's hoax hospital, once again a luxury destination, is known as "America's Most Haunted Hotel." It is said to be haunted by at least eight spirits. Its few years as a cancer hospital contributed amply to the hauntings.

A phantom nurse in white pushes a ghostly gurney on the third floor. This is an area of the building that housed Baker's morgue. Today, when a body is seen on the gurney, it means someone has died at the hotel.

Theodora continually returns from the floor below to her room on the fourth floor when it is being cleaned. Her ghost thanks the housekeeper, says that she is a patient, lies down on the freshly made bed, and disappears.

In 2005, an investigation of the hotel by television personalities Jason Hawes and Grant Wilson was produced as an episode of *Ghost Hunters*. Using a thermal-imaging camera, Wilson recorded a full-body apparition of a man who was otherwise invisible. The ghost may be one of several at the Crescent Hotel who have never been documented. Theodora, on the other hand, is seen in her entirety and speaks politely to whoever is in her room when she first appears.

Surrounded by acres of formal gardens and nature trails, the fully restored hotel provides a dozen luxury suites and a large number of guest rooms, many with their own balconies and dramatic mountain views. Of course, the most exciting view might be standing right behind guests when they're inside the Crescent Hotel.

Management currently offers nightly ghost tours, which include a visit to Baker's morgue. Visitors never know who they might run into. Some have seen flashes of purple, most often a shade of lavender, accompanying the figure of a ghost man with white hair standing outside rooms on the third floor.

OTHER ARKANSAS SIGHTINGS

BENTON

At Saline Memorial Hospital in Benton, a malodorous ghost moves into any unoccupied patient room and literally smells up the place. A voice that may be that of the ghost is heard to ask for help from inside a room. When the door is opened, a hideous odor ensues. If the door is not closed quickly enough, the foul smell moves into the hallway. The housekeeping department is called and an employee dispatched. By the time the housekeeper arrives, the smell is gone.

An old man named Ragsdale died in the hospital years ago. A hospital staffer believes the malodorous assaults are simply Mr. Ragsdale wanting someone to pull his finger. While it's unclear what he's been eating, one hopes the ghost's odoriferous finger joke is not infectious.

FORREST CITY

Originally a doctor's clinic built in 1906, the Rush-Gates House is now the home of the St. Francis County Museum. The building with a wraparound columned porch served as the home and medical practice of J. O. Rush until the surgeon's death in 1961. While rumors that the house is filled with the walking ghosts of those maimed, injured, and killed in a railroad accident may be just that, shadowy figures are seen inside the building at night when it is otherwise vacant and locked.

The persistence of ghost sightings from outside the house led the museum to invite in a paranormal research team, which documented several accounts of physical contact by ghosts. Though unseen from inside the house, the touchy ghosts appear eager to engage in shaking hands and the occasional slap on the back. The director of the museum also notes that, during the day, things tend to disappear and, when sought, appear somewhere else in the building.

For those who don't mind being poked, the museum offers to the public an annual night of ghost investigation.

FORT SMITH

Elvis Presley received his first military haircut at Fort Chaffee, located adjacent to the town of Fort Smith. Originally constructed along the Arkansas River in 1941, the military facilities grew to include an 834-bed hospital, an emergency room, operating rooms, an obstetrics facility, and dental offices. Fires have destroyed many of the buildings, and the hospital grounds and the remaining structures have been abandoned.

Someone, however, was left behind. Thought to have been a ghost when the fires took their toll, an army dentist is said to jealously guard his treatment chair, now charred, in one of the burnt buildings. Already dead and haunting his former place of practice, the ghost did not flee from the building when it burned. Trapped perhaps by his dedication to dentistry, the ghost is thoroughly toasted, if not an outright hunk of burning love.

Accounts of ghost activity at the grounds suggest that the well-roasted ghost has tired of waiting for someone to sit in his chair and that he wanders at night, looking for teeth to pull or drill. Most recently caught in car headlights, the dentist appears to have glowing red rings around his eyes. Some believe the specter may have been sporting a pair of glasses when he died.

HARRISBURG

Recently, the Harrisburg High School choir performed at the old Verser Clinic Hospital, a two-story brick building on East Street. As the lights darkened, a few of those attending yelped and jumped from their chairs. Members of the audience, one after another, reportedly came in contact with a ghost, believed to be a former patient at Verser. The building, once a Baptist church, is best remembered as the medical clinic and hospital of Dr. Joe Verser and his partner, Dr. Forrester.

Several students reported being pushed to the limit by ghost activities while helping set up the event. Two were so thoroughly frightened that they left their work unfinished and refused to return. Students said that doors closed mysteriously and locked them inside the old hospital rooms. This could have been pranking pulled off by nimble high-school students. However, once the students were trapped, with no one else present, the real ghost activity began. One student reported being held briefly by the upper arm and rubbed there, as though someone were preparing to give her an injection. She believed the experience was an encounter with Dr. Verser, who was carrying on his life's work from beyond the grave.

Later reports of paranormal research teams investigating the site have emphasized that something otherworldly is going on at Verser Clinic Hospital. A few locals return to the old hospital now and then when they want a shot at seeing a doctor without an appointment.

HOT SPRINGS

The Arkansas Rehabilitation Center in Hot Springs, originally constructed as Army-Navy Hospital, is the home of numerous hauntings. Built in 1931, the massive Art Deco structure dominates the hill overlooking the old downtown. From 1941 to 1945, more than fourteen thousand soldiers were treated at the hospital. In later years, the building was used to provide treatment for the criminally insane. Other patients suffering dementia while incarcerated by the state were relocated to the facility.

During its tenure as an institution for the mentally ill, the facility experienced many inmate deaths. The ghosts of those who died are said to inhabit the walls of two upper-story rooms where bodies were stored until they could be sent elsewhere. While some of the dead are known to speak in whispers and mumbles, the dead in this part of the old Army-Navy Hospital are a bit more vocal. Their cries for help, emerging from the plaster walls, are heard only as the doors of the elevator adjacent to the rooms open and close.

It has been suggested that the towering building might be cleansed of these haunted souls by opening the doors to the rooms and allowing the vociferous spirits to descend on the elevator.

MENA

Founded during the building of the Kansas City, Pittsburg and Gulf Railroad, Mena was settled and incorporated in 1896, the same year train service began. At about that time, Benjamin Shaver built a large home on Twelfth Street. Originally surrounded by an orchard, the Victorian two-and-a-half-story became Mena's first hospital in the 1930s and later Mena General Hospital. Now operated as an inn, the residence boasts a five-section second-story porch supported by Ionic columns.

The upper floor of the house is haunted by the ghost of a young girl who died while being treated for burns suffered in a house fire in Mena. She walks the porch late at night, apparently looking for a way home. The ghost is unable to leave the porch, perhaps because the house she seeks to go home to burned to the ground in the fire.

PARAGOULD

The ghost of a nameless boy in striped pajamas and socks walks silently in and out of patient rooms on the fourth floor of Arkansas Methodist Medical Center in Paragould. The youngster is always seen clutching a book to his chest. Estimated to be no more than five years old, the boy appears to be looking for someone to read him a bedtime story. A recent report included the detail that when the book is opened, the pages are blank.

PINE BLUFF

Davis Hospital, established in 1910, moved to a new location on Forty-second Street in Pine Bluff and was later renamed Jefferson Memorial. Having expanded several times over the years, it is now Jefferson Regional Medical Center, the city's largest employer. The original Davis Hospital was demolished in 2009. Nothing of it remains—except for one dedicated former employee who now practices her profession in the modern patient rooms at Jefferson Regional.

Some ghosts prefer to keep themselves anonymous. The nurse who migrated from the fallen bricks of the old Davis Hospital is one of them.

She never shows her face. In fact, she is so adept at it that staff members at Jefferson Regional refer to her as "the Nurse with No Face." She routinely appears in the hospital rooms of patients scheduled for surgery the next day. Her appearance portends that a patient's surgery will be successful.

FLORIDA

HOSPITAL FOR ONE
PHILLIPS MAUSOLEUM, OAKLAND CEMETERY,
838 NORTH BRONOUGH STREET,
TALLAHASSEE

IN EARLY 1919, Calvin C. Phillips triggered the latching mechanism inside the coffin. The lid lifted. One side of the polished wooden box fell away on silent hinges. The cherry-wood coffin, designed by Phillips, worked marvelously. The mechanics, like those of the clock tower attached to the retired architect's home in Tallahassee, Florida, would not rust.

"How long was I dead this time?" he asked, reaching for his cane.

"One hour, seventeen minutes, thirty-two seconds," his friend replied.

"It's getting worse, then," Phillips said. The clock chiming above him usually brought him out of his catatonic stupors.

His confidant, the local mortician and of late his only friend, simply nodded.

"We better go to the mausoleum," Phillips suggested. There, he had a casket much like this one, though the mechanism was a little different. The mausoleum was designed as both treatment room for Phillips's peculiar affliction and as his final resting place.

Phillips was a retired architect of some prominence, having been selected to design structures for the 1878 World's Fair in Paris. A noted contributor to the *Gazette des Beaux Arts* and the *American Art Journal*, Phillips excelled at design.

Late in life, recurring bouts of depression and panic began to manifest as states of brief catatonic stupor. Frightened he might mistakenly be buried alive as the durations of his coma-like stupors lengthened, Phil-

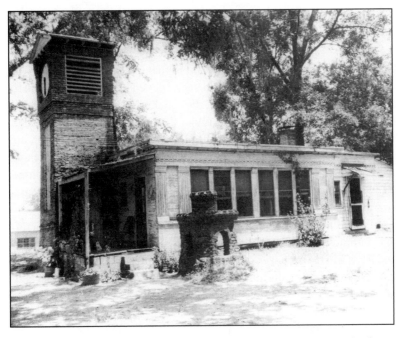

Clock tower and the Phillips home at 815 South Macomb Street in Tallahassee, Florida
STATE ARCHIVES OF FLORIDA, FLORIDA MEMORY

lips left his family. While his estranged wife and two daughters lived in
New York, he sought solitude in 1907 in Tallahassee, where he built an
architecturally unique private residence with an adjoining clock tower
designed to resemble an Arts and Crafts pendulum clock. Working clock
hands noted the hours and minutes on the exterior of the odd structure.

Inside was his casket room.

The old man discovered once he moved to Florida that he also suffered from recurrent sleep paralysis that occurred upon the conclusion of
his episodes of catatonia. The sleep paralysis was worse than the stupor.
As the architect slowly regained consciousness, he found he was unable
to function physically but was fully aware of his surroundings. He would

attempt to move his arms and legs but couldn't. These periods intensified the panic.

Like the catatonic states, his episodes of the dreaded paralysis were brief in the beginning. They were no more than mere moments. But over the years, as his beard grew and he became dependent on using a cane to stay upright, the wakeful paralysis at the conclusion of his catatonic slumbers increased significantly. Alone under the soft clucking of the wooden gears in his clock tower, Phillips would lie trapped in a state of horrific and total paralysis, each second of which was nearly unbearable. To quell the heinous and execrable horror of being locked in place, he focused on the sounds above him. The rhythm of his clock became the old man's heartbeat.

Fearful that others would take advantage of him when he fell victim to catatonic stupors and recurring paralysis, Phillips lived in isolation in Tallahassee. He was never once seen visiting the post office or the bank. Other than working on his buildings, he spent his spare time checking his watch as his beard grew longer and longer. Worried he might not die there if he left the property, the aged architect stayed home as much as he possibly could.

And he worried about a more gruesome outcome. Being buried in the ground during an extended catatonic stupor, when others might think he was dead, and waking inside a box underground, at the mercy of darkness and worms, was not a situation he intended to endure. So Phillips befriended the local undertaker and set out to erect his home of the future, a mausoleum at Oakland Cemetery. With a bed inside for his recovery from a catatonic stupor that might be mistaken for death, the mausoleum would serve as both a resting place and a final resting place. Whichever came first.

When completed, the domed mausoleum housed one of his trick-latch coffins. It was the first mausoleum constructed at Oakland Cemetery.

"Here," he said, "you keep this." Phillips handed a key to the lock on the mausoleum door to the mortician.

They stepped inside.

"Press here and then here," Phillips said. He set aside his cane and demonstrated how the casket side dropped open when the latch was manipulated from the outside. "If the casket is closed, I'm inside and will need fresh air to recover fully."

The retired architect climbed slowly into the open casket to demonstrate its fit and comfort.

"Now, close it for me."

A chill ran up the mortician's back. The gentleman had seen many dead people in his caskets. He'd put them there. A living person, though, was an altogether different experience, and a frightening one. But he did as requested, bringing the side up and latching the lid. He looked at his watch.

Soon, the casket popped open and Phillips awkwardly, painfully climbed out. He was almost smiling. Everything he'd set out to have in place in case of a misdiagnosed death was accomplished.

"Now, if I'm not in the casket, I'll be here waiting on you." With his cane, Phillips poked the recovery bed next to the casket. "Some fool will have brought me here without my key to the door."

"You should wear the key on your person," the undertaker suggested.

"I'll be sure it stays there."

"And what if you are on holiday or have taken ill? Someone else might remove it."

The mortician acknowledged that this possibility shouldn't be overlooked. He scrutinized his companion's long white whiskers and clouded eyes. His spine was permanently curved. The old man's hands and face trembled. The cane was a necessity. It wouldn't be long before the retired architect was here in his mausoleum for the ages.

"Either way," Phillips continued, lifting the cover on the bed to reveal what was underneath, "I have water for several days, a chamber pot, and three different tonics for a quick and sturdy recovery from any resulting torpor or lethargy."

They exited the mausoleum. Though small, it was most impressive.

The four outer corners were outfitted with Doric columns topped with sculpted pineapples. Higher up, turrets surrounded the base of the dome, which itself was reminiscent of the Taj Mahal.

The Tallahassee mortician turned his key in the lock.

"If you're here and a day passes, come inside and wind my watch," Phillips said.

Phillips hobbled home on his cane, his free arm held tightly across his chest like the hand of a clock.

A month later, the mortician walked by the mausoleum and noticed the door was open. He looked inside. The old man in his long white beard sat on the bed.

"Last night's episode was almost two hours," Phillips said. "I was awake at one point but couldn't move a muscle, not even my eyes."

"What did you do?"

"I listened to the clock. Being in the tower room is like sleeping inside of one." The old man coughed. His body shook. "Oh, and I have a new elixir. It's here under the bed with the others. I tried it out. It's got quite a kick."

The undertaker nodded.

"The caskets are cherry wood, did I tell you that?"

"Yes, sir, you did," the mortician replied.

"And I gave another key to the mausoleum to William Hodges, my attorney."

"Everything seems to be in order, then," the mortician said.

When he dropped by the mausoleum in the middle of November, he again found the door open. This time, Calvin C. Phillips was dead. He was on his back on the recovery bed, the casket tripped open at his side. His cane was flat on the floor.

The mortician checked his watch. "It's 2:45 P.M., Calvin."

A few moments later, he closed and locked the mausoleum and sent a message to William Hodges.

The next day, he learned there would be no funeral service for his friend. The local authorities closed the house to discourage trespassers.

The wooden gears in the clock tower soon stopped working. Over the decades, the house fell to ruin. The furniture was removed by thieves. Vandals defaced the walls inside. The tower last stood in the 1970s, before crumbling to pieces on the ground; the spare casket was long since stolen.

About the time the tower clock stopped working, people who ventured by the mausoleum began noting that they felt someone who wasn't physically there tug at their sleeves. As if to look at the watch underneath.

Someone stole Calvin C. Phillips's skull from the mausoleum. A heavy lock and hasp were added to the door of the little gem of a building, now blackened by the years.

It doesn't much matter that Phillips no longer has a head. His is a ghost you'll never see. You'll simply feel a tug upon your sleeve when walking past the Phillips mausoleum in Oakland Cemetery. Or perhaps you'll feel your wrist being turned to expose the face of your watch.

How long has he been dead this time?

Ninety-five years, Mr. Phillips. And counting.

ALL IN
BILTMORE HOTEL,
1200 ANASTASIA AVENUE,
CORAL GABLES

IT WAS GETTING NEAR DAWN on March 4, 1929. Only two players held cards at the table. Mobster Thomas "Fatty" Walsh folded his final hand to a large raise, signaling the end of a ten-hour poker marathon on the thirteenth floor of the Coral Gables Biltmore.

"What you got?" he asked the victor, growling the question to the side of a burning cigar clamped in his teeth.

"Nothing much," local gambler Eddie Wilson replied. Wilson leased the entire thirteenth floor of the grand hotel and operated it as an illegal but popular speakeasy and gambling hall during Prohibition.

Fatty Walsh didn't care what was gilt and what was marble. He didn't care how tall the fountain was in the ground-floor lobby. As far as he was concerned, a pocketful of poker chips defined the lap of luxury. In his world, *grand* meant a thousand dollars, and you showed your cards when you won a hand.

"Show me," Fatty said. The New York gangster, a recent transplant to Florida, was a well-known associate of Dutch Schultz and Lucky Luciano. He expected any request he made to be followed. Quickly.

Eddie had other plans. He replaced his cards face down into the middle of deck, enraging the volatile Walsh. Fatty came to his feet in a single surge, kicking over his chair and shoving his arms and shoulders across the poker table.

Eddie shot him in mid-lunge. The gangster fell dead, his chips cashed in. His hat and cigar tumbled to the floor.

"Move his body and put out the cigar," Eddie instructed his employees. "Clean this place up and call the cops. Tell them he started it."

The epitome of the Roaring Twenties, the palatial Coral Gables Biltmore opened in 1926 and set the pace for live entertainment, legal and otherwise. Thousands attended the weekend aquatic galas at the hotel, which included synchronized swimmers, bathing beauties, and alligator wrestling. Four-year-old sensation Jackie Ott stunned the crowds by diving from an eighty-five-foot platform into the hotel pool. Prior to his Hollywood yodeling and lion-wrestling days as Tarzan, Johnny Weissmuller, a gold-medal winner at the 1924 and 1928 summer Olympics, was a swimming instructor at the Biltmore.

On the grand terrace, swing bands played the latest ragtime, foxtrots, and tangos. Flappers in jewels and oiled-hair hipsters in tuxedos made their way around a cascading two-story fountain in the courtyard of the ballroom, strolling under gilt-detailed arched ceilings held aloft by marbles columns. Among numerous notable guests at the lavish Biltmore were the Duke and Duchess of Windsor and a variety of Vanderbilts. Fred Astaire, Ginger Rogers, Judy Garland, and Bing Crosby could be seen from time to time in the lobby. Al Capone had a favorite room there. So did Franklin D. Roosevelt, who maintained a temporary White House office in the hotel while vacationing in the area.

The bombing of Pearl Harbor changed the world. The fabulous hotel was no exception. In 1942, as American automakers switched to building tanks, Jeeps, and airplanes, the federal government took control of the Coral Gables Biltmore. Uncle Sam repurposed the grand hotel into a hospital for American servicemen wounded in battle. In the process, many of the windows were sealed with concrete. Marble floors were covered with government-issued linoleum. Guest rooms became patient rooms, and a morgue was built inside the structure.

But a war doesn't end poker.

During those years of service to the war effort, nurses spoke among themselves of the always-present smell of cigar smoke on the private elevator to the thirteenth floor. Men were heard playing poker in rooms that turned out to be empty. The sound of poker chips being counted, stacked, and dispersed went away when the doors to vacant rooms were opened by curious hospital staff.

"Everyone who worked there visited the thirteenth floor just to hear what was going on," a retired army nurse reported. "They said it was Fatty Walsh still shuffling and dealing cards more than twelve years after he was shot dead in one of the rooms after losing a poker game."

Converted to Army Air Forces Regional Hospital, the once-opulent Biltmore remained a medical facility long after the war. Until 1968, it served as both a VA hospital and the medical school of the University of Miami. Through it all, Fatty Walsh kept dealing cards to himself and a gathering of servicemen whose most recent residence had been the morgue. A "dead man's hand" for those players wasn't aces and eights. It was any cards they happened to be holding.

In 1987, the city of Coral Gables supervised the full restoration of the original hotel at an estimated cost of $55 million. The Coral Gables Biltmore reopened as a luxury hotel and resort. Fatty Walsh was pleased. He had little use for doctors and nurses. And dead soldiers didn't have much money. Paying guests were a better deal by far.

The smell of cigar smoke lingers in the tower elevator. The sound of chips being stacked and cards being played is still heard on the thirteenth floor. Guests may sit in, if they find the right room at the right time. All they need do is knock on the door and show some money.

Today's players are advised, though, to follow the house rules. All winning hands must be shown when another player folds. And no guns are allowed.

FAIR WARNING
FORT WALTON BEACH MEDICAL CENTER,
1000 MAR-WALT DRIVE,
FORT WALTON BEACH

SOME YEARS AGO, Janie Roush sat in the backseat of her father's car and brushed her hair. Then she screamed, and soon she was dead.

It was dusk one evening in October 1972, the day after Janie's birthday, when Walter Roush picked up his daughter in the family's white Corvair from her weekly piano lesson. He asked her, smiling, if she'd decided what she wanted to do when she grew up.

"You should know, now that you're fifteen," he said, winking in the rearview mirror as he pulled the car away from the curb.

Janie did not reply.

"She wants to be famous," her little brother said. He rode in the passenger seat up front.

"Being famous isn't something you do," Walter said.

If they didn't shut up about it, Janie was going to scream.

She screamed anyway, just after Walter mistakenly piloted the car through a busy intersection in Fort Walton Beach after the light had changed. A Ford van T-boned the lightweight car on the passenger side, crushing and instantly killing Janie's brother. The impact threw Walter from the collapsing rear-engine Corvair. He discovered death the moment his head slammed into the pavement. Broken glass filled the front and back seats as Janie's screams filled the night air.

The broken radiator in the van hissed. A piece of chrome stuck into Janie's upper abdomen. Her collarbone had snapped in two when her shoulder was slammed against the inside of the car. Janie seemed to occupy a world that spun around her where she lay sideways in the backseat, in fear and pain. She screamed and screamed some more, swallowing two tiny pieces of broken glass as she did. The lining of her throat was cut. Blood ran from her forehead, clouding her vision.

Janie's high-pitched screams turned hoarse, then faded. Soon, all she could manage were a few shallow breaths and a burning rasp as she struggled to understand what had happened and what was happening still.

The wail of sirens replaced her screams. The night was painted by flashing red lights as two men lifted Janie from the car. Her long, shiny hair was matted with blood. She was alive when they placed her in the ambulance, but her prognosis was grim. Janie died just outside the emergency-room entrance at Fort Walton Beach Medical Center.

The pain disappeared. No more alive than a stone, decorated by blood and damaged flesh, Janie climbed off the gurney and walked away. Exiting the parking area, she worried that her hair was a mess. Janie set out to find her brush. It was, she believed, still in the car. As she walked, the teenager maintained flawless posture that showed off her long, straight hair to its best advantage. She noticed, however, that the ragged piece of chrome ruined the front of her sweater.

Scared and dead, she pressed her fingers to her throat and tried to scream. And scream she did, loud and shrill. Her throat, at least, worked again. She screamed one more time to make sure.

Janie's goal in life at age fifteen had been to be famous. As she walked, she reconsidered how that might best occur now that she was no longer in school. She could play piano and sing. She wasn't much of an actress, but she could walk like a model. And she could scream. That made four things, along with having gorgeous blond hair.

The crushed Corvair was still at the intersection when she arrived. Police cars blocked off traffic. The van with the crunched front end was nearby. An officer walked a measuring wheel from here to there and made entries in a flip-top notebook. People who had parked their cars or come running from nearby doorways gathered to view the wreckage. Someone was taking pictures with a flash camera.

Janie held her shoulders up and strode to the Corvair. She located her hairbrush on the floor, in front of the seat where she'd been primly sitting a short time earlier.

Her brother and father were dead. She was, too. Fatality was a big step in her life, for sure. She wondered, *Now what?* There had to be something she could do.

She walked back to the emergency-room parking lot and stared at the parked ambulances. Janie rubbed her eyes with the back of her hand to clear her vision of blood. Whatever she did now was what she was going to be when she grew up, Janie realized. She'd grown up as far as she was going to.

It wasn't long, or it might have been a day or two, when she watched an ambulance leave the parking lot, its siren wailing as it turned on to the street. Janie knew at that moment what she would do for the rest of her time on planet earth. However long that might be. The fifteen-year-old could fill a need and become famous for it.

There were no sirens before car accidents. Only after. It didn't do the people in wrecked cars much good at all. Plain and simple, there should be sirens before a wreck.

Janie walks the neighborhoods in Fort Walton Beach. People in violent accidents say that, just before the incident occurs, they hear a scream that sounds like a woman's. Janie Roush, dead since 1972, is still working on her timing. So far as anyone has reported, she hasn't stopped a wreck from happening.

But non-wrecks, after all, don't make the news. Most go unreported. Perhaps the people she saves from catastrophe pause to take a deep breath and thank their lucky stars before driving on.

The drivers should thank Janie. She's the girl in the rearview mirror with blond hair and a piece of chrome in the middle of her sweater, the girl who is about to be famous. Listen.

OTHER FLORIDA SIGHTINGS

AUBURNDALE

Good Shepherd Hospice, on the shore of Lake Ariana, is the home away from home of Mary Morrow, a ghost noted for her pleasant hospitality to patients and visitors alike. She is seen on the premises wearing a floral-print dress and is believed to be the deceased wife of a doctor who once worked at the facility.

COCONUT GROVE

A girl in glowing white is seen late at night from the upper floors of Mercy Hospital. The ghost is often viewed walking the soccer field of the adjacent La Salle High School, on the shore of Biscayne Bay. A rare example of a point-of-view ghost, the girl cannot be seen from either outside the hospital or from La Salle High School itself.

CORAL SPRINGS

A nurse who worked at Coral Springs Medical Center was brought to the emergency room and died there.

She continues to work at the center even today, although the only thing she seems to remember about being an R.N. is giving shots. She does so painlessly. Her chosen patients report that they feel the needle going in and being pulled out, but that it doesn't hurt. They feel only a tingle.

The ghost nurse, however, doesn't give shots in the arm. Sometimes call "the Bottoms Up Ghost," the needle-happy nurse waits until patients roll over in bed and are lying on their side.

DELAND

The original DeLand Memorial Hospital, listed on the National Register of Historic Places, currently houses a local-history museum. Ex-

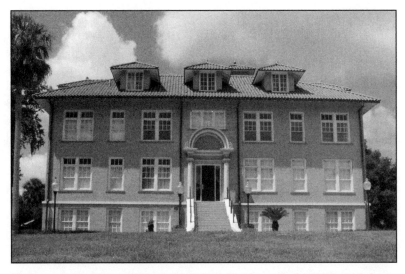

The former DeLand Memorial Hospital in Deland, Florida, was built in 1920 and dedicated to the veterans of World War I. The building is currently the DeLand Memorial Hospital Museum. UNIVERSITY OF NORTH FLORIDA

hibits include a 1920s operating room, a rare apothecary display, and a gallery of memorabilia. A smaller structure behind DeLand Memorial, the Burgess Building, provided surgical and obstetrical services for local African-Americans.

Both sites are haunted by the ghosts of former patients who walk the grounds, apparently returning from where they were buried to the location of their final breaths. Once gathered in groups, the specters are often mistaken for zombies. The walking ghosts first appear as face-sized fog on the windows of parked cars. Soon, hands appear alongside as the faces take shape. Additional faces and hands appear unless and until the ghosts are abruptly disturbed by a car horn or by shouts from inside the vehicle. It was recently documented that a scream will suffice. More disturbingly, local residents report that ghosts on their way to the hospital are seen strolling through occupied houses in DeLand.

JACKSONVILLE

A suite of medical offices at 915 West Monroe Street was built near the site of George A. Brewster Hospital, erected to treat victims of the great fire in Jacksonville in 1901, considered one of the worst disasters in Florida history and the largest urban fire in the southeastern United States. The conflagration began in the middle of a workday on May 3 when a boiler exploded at a candle factory, causing a fire that spread to a mattress factory, setting ablaze mattresses filled with the South's famed Spanish moss.

The fire burned 146 city blocks, destroyed more than 2,300 buildings, and left approximately 10,000 residents homeless. The glow from the flames could be seen in Savannah, Georgia, and the smoke plumes were visible as far away as Raleigh, North Carolina. For years following the fire, visitors said they could smell Jacksonville before they saw it.

Brewster Hospital soon expanded to include a school for training nurses. The original building was recently moved and is being preserved. The location, however, remains haunted by former patients of the hospital. The ghosts walk from unknown locations on their way to the hospital. According to residents, the ghosts appear soon after the scent of something burning.

ORLANDO

The former Sunland Mental Hospital in the Pine Hills section of Orlando has been demolished and is now a park. The facility specialized in the treatment and housing of children with severe mental handicaps. It closed in 1983 amid charges of abuse and neglect. Not to mention the rats. Considered an unsafe structure, the hospital was torn down fifteen years later. During that time, it became popular as a place to hear, if not see, ghosts.

Swimming was by far the most popular activity for patients at Sunland. The pool was one of the good things at the hospital. Ramps and rails were installed in the shallow end. Otherwise immobilized children rolled into the water in their wheeled swimming chairs. The noise of children playing in the pool was at times deafening.

After the hospital closed, those who visited the abandoned facility reported hearing splashing and the sounds of children playing in the now-empty pool.

The pool was filled in and buried when the building was razed. The resulting park is a level area of carefully mown grass among a few surviving trees. No signs of a hospital remain on the old Sunland site. None that can be seen. However, the sounds of bodies jumping into water and splashing in the pool, along with the accompanying laughter and screeches of children at play, can still be heard by those who walk through the park.

Children know what they like best. They return from the afterlife to a pool that isn't there to relive their grandest activity and have a good time again. For some children, at least, having been housed—and likely mistreated—at Sunland Mental Hospital means they get to swim and play for eternity.

PENSACOLA

The original Sacred Heart Hospital on Twelfth Street, also known as Old Pensacola Hospital, was the first Catholic hospital in Florida and is listed on the National Register of Historic Places. Built in 1915, the Gothic Revival multistory stone structure is both a medical and architectural landmark.

It's also a landmark to the unending services of a deceased hospital sister who frequents the hallway just outside the old chapel. Voices in the hallway can be heard inside the chapel. People who are talking in the hallway experience the ghostly nun as a tap or two on the shoulder to remind them to be quiet.

PENSACOLA

The main education and training building at Corry Station Naval Technical Training Center was completed in 1834, a few years after President John Quincy Adams assigned surgeon Isaac Hulse to establish a hospital at the Pensacola Navy Yard. The structure served as a hospital through 1985. Numerous servicemen who succumbed to yellow fever in the 1830s were interred at nearby Barrancas Cemetery, long in use as a burial ground and formally established as a United States naval cemetery in 1838.

Ghosts from both the hospital and the cemetery are active in the old hospital building. Appearing as wisps of fog, the dead are noted for flinging objects across rooms and for writing messages on the walls that warn of impending death. It is unclear whom they intend to warn. Some suggest the dire messages are meant for those treated at the hospital during yellow-fever outbreaks. Others believe the ghosts are seeking to capture the attention of the living.

If so, they're doing a good job of it.

SARASOTA

Sarasota Memorial Hospital, a regional medical center in the heart of Florida's famed circus country, is haunted by a specter known as "the Melting Ghost." The ghost of a circus performer is often seen in the doorways of patient rooms. The dead clown's makeup is not holding up well in the afterlife. In fact, it's a runny mess. The ghost clown's smile appears to those who see him to be melting.

It is said the performer died of a fever that caused his makeup to run.

ST. AUGUSTINE

The Spanish Military Hospital Museum, a reconstruction of Our Lady of Guadalupe Hospital, is beset by a notable haunting. A man of short stature dashes from room to room. Dressed in brown, he quickly appears and disappears, all the while swinging a hatchet over his head.

The vision began to appear as a new water line was being laid at the hospital site, when workers excavated an ancient internment of human bones—a burial ground of the indigenous Timucua Indians. The oldest bones dated to the arrival of Europeans in the New World. Warfare with the British ended the Timucua, who became extinct in the early 1800s.

The man dressed in brown at the St. Augustine hospital museum is believed to have risen when his bones were disturbed. Lurching from room to room with a hatchet, he certainly appears to be mad at somebody.

WINTER PARK

The eighty-year-old Annie Russell Theatre on the campus of Rollins College in Winter Park is inhabited by the ghost of Annie herself, an English-born actress who taught drama and theater at the school until her death in 1936.

Annie is also referred to as "Doctor Annie" by a kindly few, although she had no medical training whatsoever. The nickname was earned by the actions of the actress/director when a young man was injured at her theater. And by the recurring actions of her ghost.

Late at night, when the theater is dark, a male voice is heard to call out, "The ambulance is here!" Upon this announcement, Annie appears in 1930s clothing and jumps into action. She hurriedly ushers two ambulance attendants into the theater and reappears on stage to attend to an injured young man lying there. Soon, the attendants join her. With care, they load the crumpled body onto a hospital gurney. As they exit the theater, Annie holds open the doors for them.

City records indicate that an ambulance was dispatched to the Annie Russell Theatre to assist a young man who fell while working on the lights above the stage. Oddly, this incident occurred more than twenty-five years after Annie passed away.

Annie Russell, though dead, continues to direct emergency care. For her, the show . . . and life . . . must go on. And on. For at least as long as her theater is standing.

GEORGIA

GOT YOUR NOSE
OLD MEDICAL COLLEGE OF GEORGIA, 598 TELFAIR STREET, AUGUSTA

NESTLED AMONG THE TALL TREES on Telfair Street in Augusta is a handsome old building with an impressive portico of six Doric columns supporting a classical triangular pediment. It is believed to be haunted by as many as four hundred ghosts.

One night during the pre–Civil War years, the dean of the Medical College of Georgia carried a lantern to a wagon that had drawn to a stop behind the school. A slave hurried to the back of the plantation wagon to uncover his goods, which were neatly tucked beneath a spread of canvas. As the black man pulled back the canvas, the dean lifted his lantern and examined the two corpses.

"Both from the same place?"

"Yes, sir."

"This one's no good," the dean complained. "Been dead too long, and he's too parched. The muscle may as well be boards, and the organs are folded in. You can tell from the eyes. They look like burnt raisins. I can't take it. Bury him somewhere."

The dean moved his lantern to scrutinize the smaller body. He lifted the arm and let it fall.

"How old is she?"

"Seven, sir. Right at seven. Ate wild berries that were poison."

The dean paid seventy-five cents, which the slave would take to his master. He set down his lantern. There had to be a better way, the dean thought.

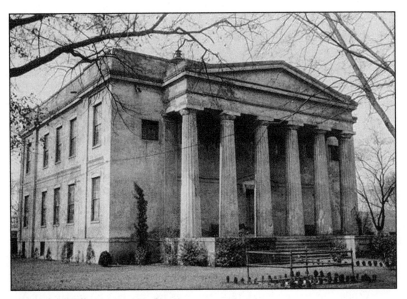

Old Medical College in Augusta, Georgia
HISTORIC AMERICAN BUILDINGS SURVEY

And there was. The better way turned out to be a thirty-six-year-old slave the dean purchased for seven hundred dollars on a trip to Charleston in 1852. West African–born Grandison Harris was brought to Augusta and given exceptionally fine quarters in the basement of the medical college. The slave's pregnant wife remained in Charleston. Grandison had no choice in the matter.

Grandison's duties at the college encompassed a little bit of everything. He moved chairs and tables and benches. He groomed and fed the dean's horses. He carried anything heavy that needed to be carried. And he ran errands.

"Get to know the Negroes around town," the dean instructed him. "Go to the Baptist church in Springfield and learn their names and meet their families. And here on Greene Street, the ones that are working."

The dean showed him everything, barking from the back of his carriage while Grandison snapped the reins to have the horse turn a corner, and another one. Eventually, they came to Boundary Street. Then the dean gave directions to Cedar Grove Cemetery.

"There's someone here I want you to meet."

Grandison was taught to wash his teeth and hands at least once a day, to bathe on Saturdays, to go to church on Sundays, and to learn the words of the Bible and the hymns. He was also taught to read the newspaper. It was against the law to teach a slave to read, but the dean and his fellow doctors allowed themselves the privilege.

And one more thing. Grandison was taught to retrieve recently deceased bodies and bring them to the medical college.

The outbreak of war in 1861 curtailed operations at the college. Faculty of the right age and students withdrew their participation in medical education to serve in the Confederate army. Cadavers weren't needed. Grandison performed his other duties and concentrated on learning to read more sophisticated books. He learned all the stories in the Bible.

When the war ended, Grandison was no longer a slave. He left Augusta but returned to the medical college shortly afterward, bringing with him his wife and son. She'd named the boy George, after America's first president. The dean hired Grandison and paid him eight dollars monthly to serve as the school's porter.

But what he carried to and fro wasn't luggage. Grandison developed a regular source for fresh bodies. No one cared to ask for details. The Medical College of Georgia soon boasted, among its achievements in medicine, the finest anatomy specimens in the South.

Everyone seemed to know what was going on, but not officially. It wasn't something a gentleman said out loud. Students at the college nicknamed Grandison "the Resurrection Man."

The African-American community had other words to describe him. Black children in Augusta were warned that Grandison would come for them in the middle of the night if they misbehaved.

"Grandy got your nose," an uncle told his niece, placing his fingers on either side of her nose and giving a tug before pulling his hand away and hiding it behind him.

The little girl said to give it back.

"When Grandison takes your nose, he's not leaving the rest of you behind, you can count on that," the uncle said. "He gets your nose and toes and everything in between."

Grandison Harris retired in 1908. The Medical College of Georgia, in need of larger facilities, moved to a new location. The original building, after serving a number of purposes and providing space to a variety of organizations, underwent extensive renovation in 1989. That was when the ghosts, long since settled into their home at the old medical college, woke up.

Workers removing the floor in what was now a kitchen found a bone. Another bone was quickly revealed. The authorities were called. Both bones were human.

The floor of the basement sat on top of a bunch of bones—dozens of old bones and dozens more. A few were marked with specimen numbers. The basement appeared to be a dumping ground for bones.

Human bones were found by the bucket. And not only by the bucket, but in a bucket. A lidded vat the size of a barrel held human bones that appeared to have been boiled. Another old vat contained human body parts still preserved in whiskey. By the time people stopped looking, the bones, hidden cadavers, and body parts found were judged to be the remains of between 350 and 450 people.

Experts were called in. The bones, now numbering in the thousands, were sorted, typed, and counted by Robert Blakely's forensic anthropology students at Georgia State University. More than nine thousand human bones, it turned out, were removed from the basement of the old medical college.

The ghosts came out, and so did the stories.

Grandison Harris was a body snatcher. It was said he frequently opened the graves of the recently buried at the all-black Cedar Grove Cemetery and carried the bodies in a wagon to the medical college. Grandison was so adept that he would open only one end of a grave, break into the casket, and pull the body out by their ears and nose. So skilled a graverobber did he become that he'd memorize the position of flowers above the grave and, after deftly filling the hole he'd dug, replace them exactly the same. His talent was so advanced that he made not a single sound and was never discovered. Never caught by anyone. Never seen or heard at Cedar Grove.

People in the African-American community of Augusta certainly knew, according to historians. As word spread among black citizens about the theft and use of their dead, authorities faced a civil disturbance in 1889. The use of the dead meant dissection.

"When the old folks learned about that, Augusta almost had its own riot," says James Carter III, a retired Medical College of Georgia administrator and Augusta historian. "They were so upset because they didn't know whose family members had been taken."

Taken, cut to pieces, and placed in jars. People refused to have their deceased family members buried at Cedar Grove.

It would be a hundred years later, in 1989, that proof surfaced that the community's fear was grounded in reality. More than nine thousand pieces of proof that, if Grandison got your nose, he also got your toes and everything in between.

All of the remains discovered at the old medical college were reinterred at Cedar Grove. A ceremony was held at the cemetery in 1999, and a brass plaque with a somber account of the bodies' removal was put into place. There's also some stuff there about the bodies having performed a service to mankind's understanding of anatomy and disease.

What isn't on the plaque is an acknowledgment that Grandison Harris couldn't possibly have removed that many bodies over such a long period of time without help from others. Many of the stolen bodies were likely never buried, although a large number of empty caskets probably were. It's more than feasible that a local undertaker or two was involved in holding back bodies from the grave.

Grandison was acquainted with the rumors. He knew all about the social upheaval in his community in 1889. He also knew more than anybody about how bodies came into the possession of the medical college. He passed away in 1911 and was buried at Cedar Grove Cemetery, long before the discovery of the basement full of bones.

His ghost doesn't live at the cemetery, though. Daylight hours, his spirit remains at the old medical college, declared a National Historic Landmark in 1996 and used as a conference and events center and occasionally as a venue for weddings.

Nighttime finds Grandison on a phantom wagon behind a phantom horse, roaming the residential neighborhoods to either side of East Boundary for someone's nose and toes to snatch, and everything in between. It's all he knows to do until the truth comes out that he alone didn't steal all those bodies. And that it's unfair to say he did. Until then, Grandison won't rest in his grave.

FOOTLOOSE
PROVIDENCE ACADEMY,
4575 LAWRENCEVILLE HIGHWAY,
AND
LILBURN MARSHALL HOUSE,
123 EAST BROUGHTON STREET,
SAVANNAH

NUMEROUS HOSPITALS WERE CREATED across the South during the War Between the States. At times of heavy fighting, tent hospitals were hastily erected near battlefields. Medical care at tent hospitals was also rather hasty, and amputations were common. Removed limbs were disposed of expediently.

Such was the case in Lilburn, Georgia. The tent hospital came and went. The sawn-off limbs, however, were left—one might say right and left—behind.

Treated as hospital waste, amputated limbs were shallowly buried in an area that is now the Spracklin-Williamson soccer field on the campus of Providence Academy. Moving ground to create a level sports field disturbed the interred limbs, which are reported to come to the surface as ghost arms and legs during soccer practice and sometimes during games. A persistent rumor that severed legs play soccer late at night has been proven to be an exaggeration. Nevertheless, the phantom limbs do at times take on physical existence. An emerging foot has been reported to trip players. An unseen hand grabs an ankle, then retreats under the grass. It is likely the limbs are reminded of battle when soccer play is under way.

Ghost limbs, if capable of possessing thought, might believe the soccer players, dressed in matching uniforms, are engaging in war. Legs and arms once trained for conflict simply can't resist. Others suggest the ghost limbs are just out for kicks.

Along with bones in the yard, it seems every old house in the South has a few skeletons in the closet. Or tucked neatly away in the attic. Or perhaps under the floor.

The oldest surviving hotel in Savannah, built in 1851 at the direction of owner Mary Marshall, has a few hidden bones of its own. The fanciful four-story structure saw duty as a Confederate hospital. It was later taken over by invading Yankees and served as a Union hospital in 1864 and 1865.

Its use as a hospital has created a number of ghosts at the Marshall House, one source of which was discovered during a multimillion-dollar renovation in 1998. While replacing floorboards on the first story, workers uncovered human bones. Upon this discovery, the immediate area was closed off as a potential crime scene. The resulting investigation quickly revealed that the only crime associated with the remains was that of war.

The room where the floorboards were being replaced had been utilized for hospital surgery during the War Between the States. The bones were amputated arms and legs.

More than one noted ghost at the Marshall House is an amputee. Guests have reported seeing a one-armed uniformed soldier wandering the lobby. A ghost with one leg has also been spotted. He offers a cavalry boot to passing hotel patrons while wearing the other one.

In Savannah, history is everywhere you look. Despite burning his way through the rest of Georgia, General William T. Sherman spared Savannah's buildings. The city is certainly blessed with a large number of original structures and more than its share of ghosts.

Some suggests Savannah's ghosts are active because of the subtropical climate. Of course, the city also has a lively history of voodoo, which might explain a few of its long-lingering ghosts. And the Spanish moss hanging from tree branches looks ghostly in and of itself. (Visitors are warned to watch out for biting ants that may infest the elegant draperies of moss.) For whatever reasons, Savannah is considered by many to be the most ghost-infested city in the South, its only competition being New Orleans.

The high probability of encountering a ghost is part of Savannah's charm. An endless parade of spooky tours of haunted mansions, streets, tunnels, cemeteries, homes, and hotels is available. Once you've caught the spellbinding stage performance of Lady Chablis, "the Empress of Savannah," at Club One on Jefferson Street, the concierge at the Marshall House will be more than happy to point you in the direction of Savannah's most popular haunts. Of course, if you're staying at the Marshall House, the ghosts are already there.

Current management readily confesses that the Marshall House is haunted. It insists, however, that most of the ghosts are friendly ambassadors of Southern hospitality—even if some are arms and legs in want of the rest of their bodies.

JUMP UP AND RUN
ANDERSONVILLE NATIONAL HISTORIC SITE, 760 POW ROAD, ANDERSONVILLE

BEING TRANSFERRED TO THE HOSPITAL was one manner of attempted escape for Union prisoners held in the deplorable conditions of the Confederate prison at Andersonville, established in February 1864. The swiftest means of exit, of course, was dying. Piles of bodies were attended to daily. The dead were loaded into body wagons and buried in mass graves. Free at last.

Once the decision was made to create a prison at Andersonville, captured Union soldiers and officers were transferred to the site in large numbers. They were held in an open-air stockade that originally encompassed sixteen and a half acres. The stockade was intended as a temporary holding area, pending exchanges of prisoners with the North. Those exchanges never happened. In June, the stockade was enlarged by an additional ten acres.

The prisoners suffered extreme lack of food, severe overcrowding, and exceedingly poor sanitary conditions. They had little drinkable water. Prisoners who weren't sick already quickly became ill at Andersonville.

Upon arriving, prisoners quickly discovered that they lacked many of life's basic necessities. Finding themselves without shelter, some constructed crude dwellings from various items including pieces of clothing, sticks, and mud bricks. Deteriorating clothing presented another problem. Some prisoners went without. Those who died late in the fourteen-month existence of Andersonville Prison were stripped and their clothes

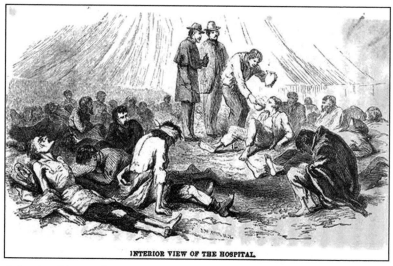

INTERIOR VIEW OF THE HOSPITAL.

A drawing of the second prison hospital in Andersonville, Georgia
NATIONAL PARK SERVICE/ANDERSONVILLE NATIONAL HISTORIC SITE

taken back inside the stockade. Historical records indicate that, on one such occasion, a prisoner's body was discovered to be female.

Availability of water was one reason the prison was established at Andersonville. A small stream, Stockade Branch, flowed through the grounds. It was the only water supply for drinking, washing clothes, and bathing. Prison latrines built on the hillside above the branch overflowed during rains, sending their contents into the water supply. Because of the severe overcrowding, there wasn't even enough contaminated water to go around.

Union prisoner John Ransom operated a barbershop inside the prison and also kept a diary. "There is so much filth about the camp that it is terrible trying to live here," he wrote. "When a spring flowed out of the ground after a heavy rainstorm and created a new water supply, the prisoners, attributing it to an act of Providence, named it Providence Spring."

The rampant sickness in Andersonville Prison soon got worse.

Although a separate area was fenced off as a hospital, prisoners suffered a dire lack of medical supplies and personnel. Following the arrival of wounded Union soldiers from the Battle of Atlanta in July 1864, Union captain Harmon Hubbard was placed in charge of specific duties at the hospital, which at that time consisted of an enclosed field with a few tents, a cook shed, and an operating table but, according to Hubbard, "no bedding, no clothing, no bandages, no medicine, and but little food." Military surgeons sawed through bones during amputations, accomplished without anesthesia.

"Many undressed wounds were fly-blown and infested with maggots," Hubbard later wrote. "Prisoners disliked being eaten by worms before death, and preferred heroic treatment with crude turpentine."

Hubbard further detailed a portion of his duties. Each morning and at various intervals during the day, he had "to drag out the dead men . . . where they could be gathered up in big wagons, from forty to fifty at a load, with six mule teams, and hauled out to the trenches, six feet wide, five feet deep and long enough to contain one thousand laid side by side, touching elbows, as in life, without coffins, shrouds or ceremonies."

Of the more than 40,000 men imprisoned at Andersonville, 13,647 are buried there.

Harmon Hubbard survived Andersonville and the war. He died in 1926. He wrote in 1904, "I do not desire to tell all that I know and remember of life and death in Andersonville. For many years I have tried to forget and cannot."

One Union soldier at Andersonville is also apparently unable to forget.

To cope with the horrible conditions, prisoners engaged in a variety of activities. They carved objects, sang songs, played checkers and cards, read any material they could get their hands on, and wrote letters home, which were censored by prison officials and seldom reached their destinations. Others intent on escape spent their time digging tunnels, although there are no records of successful escapes in that fashion.

But one soldier did escape by ingenious means in 1864. As recorded in John Ransom's diary on May 16, the prisoner spent his last day in

Andersonville Prison pretending to be dead, after which he was carried out of the main stockade and piled with the other bodies by the hospital, to await transport the next morning. Once darkness fell, he jumped up and ran for it.

The soldier's escape may not have been the first by this method, but the strategy was mimicked by other prisoners on subsequent days. Its success proved fleeting. The guards were soon alerted to the practice that became known as "the Dead Man's Run." Confederate soldiers with orders to shoot anything that moved were assigned to guard the body piles at night. From then on, prisoners who participated in the craze were shot without warning well before making it clear of rifle range.

Visitors to Andersonville National Historic Site may note that 921 graves are marked "unknown" in the cemetery there. Those who linger past dusk may also note a ghost who jumps up from the location of the body piles by the hospital site and runs for it. The ghost manages but a few leaping steps before vanishing.

OTHER GEORGIA SIGHTINGS

ATLANTA

The specialized treatment at Peachford Hospital includes therapy for addictions on both an inpatient and outpatient basis.

A former Peachford drug-rehab patient, now deceased, has swapped one addiction in life for another in the afterlife. Either that or the young man talked himself to death in the first place. The ghost's ceaseless yammering is heard late at night in the courtyard. Patients with windows overlooking the courtyard are not pleased. The loquacious ghost repeats the same stories, literally saying the same thing over and over. Ad nauseam. One patient complained, "He uses the same words and sentences every dang time. And he only talks about himself."

Sadly, treatment for ghosts with afterlife addictions is not available at Peachford at the present. And ghosts don't get better without it.

BUFORD

The construction of the Mall of Georgia brought many changes to Buford, not the least of which was the demolition of a number of closed and abandoned structures in the immediate area. The old Buford Hospital on Morningside Drive managed to escape destruction for years. The empty hospital, after being used for SWAT training, was boarded up. It sat and waited. So did the ghost of DeeAnn Parker, who died in the hospital.

An avid reader who was reliant on a wheelchair in old age, Parker found her afterlife prayers answered when the new Gwinnett County Public Library opened nearby. It was handicapped-accessible.

Parker's ghost apparently rolled her way to the library in her wheelchair. Patrons sometimes report an empty wheelchair getting in the way as Parker browses the shelves. Thus far, librarians have been unable to locate Parker herself. She's always quiet and apparently invisible. Lately, the wheelchair has been parked in front of one of the library's computers.

CLEVELAND

Residents who've come to Friendship Nursing Home to live out their lives are never thrilled to see the apparition of a young boy in a red baseball cap. This is especially true for people who believe not knowing when they're going to die is one of the best parts of life. Word among the residents is that when the boy in the red cap stands outside the door of a patient's room, it's bad news. That patient is next in line to enter the afterlife. The good news is the patient has twenty-four hours to prepare for the journey.

DOUGLASVILLE

Office employees who work beyond normal business hours at the old Douglas Hospital, now occupied by the local board of education, discover that two residents of the former hospital occupy the premises.

One is fond of writing something on a vintage typewriter. The keys are heard click-clacking away into the wee hours. Thus far, the actual typewriter has not been found.

A ghostly apparition of a nurse has been seen, but is more often heard, carrying a clinking hospital tray as she strides the halls in squeaky shoes.

DUNWOODY

The sprawling brick building that housed Brook Run Hospital in Dunwoody was left empty for a number of years before being torn down. The site has been absorbed by the adjacent city park, also known as Brook Run. The former location of the hospital is nearest the portion of the park set aside for skateboarding. Also residing there is a ghost in the ground, apparently a former patient who died at the hospital.

The leveling of the hospital site created a particular problem for the ghost. Lying on his back in bed, the ghost is now immobile, buried up to his neck in soil. And then some. The ghost appears as a circle of face in the ground. When he is stepped on, the unlucky ghost closes his eyes but doesn't make a sound.

If you're on the dog trail in Brook Run Park, you might want to keep an eye out if your four-legged companion wanders behind the concrete skateboard bowls. The ghost face so far hasn't bitten. But there's always a first time.

FORT STEWART

Fort Stewart's Winn Army Community Hospital is haunted by the ghost of a surgeon who is enamored with the modern medical equipment now in use at the facility. Wearing surgical garb that suggests he died in the 1980s, the ghost turns on medical machines in unoccupied rooms at night. The ghost also likes to keep things clean. Early in the morning, he has been spotted in the basement near the washer-sterilizer apparatus, which he turns on before fading into a rapidly dissipating fog.

MARIETTA

Built in 1845, the Kennesaw House, three stories above ground and a basement below, now houses the Marietta Museum of History. The historic building is one of the few significant antebellum structures not burned by General William T. Sherman during his March to the Sea. The general used the house as his headquarters while his soldiers set fire to much of the rest of the city.

Due to its proximity to the railroad station, the spacious structure also served as a hospital during the War Between the States. PBS, CNN, and the History Channel have aired documentaries that included the frequently repeated story of visitors who discovered a tableaux apparition of an 1860s hospital that included an amputation in progress.

More likely to be experienced today is the haunt of the building's elevator. A uniformed soldier who died while the house served as a hospital, and long before the elevator was installed, often appears when the elevator door opens. The dead soldier, many believe, is trying to ascend to heaven, but the elevator doesn't go that far.

NEWNAN

The advice to patients at Piedmont Newnan Hospital on Jackson Street was to stay in their rooms precisely at nine o'clock and feign sleep when the figure in white came by. The ghost of a former nurse was known to enter occupied patient rooms at that hour, day and night. She might come into the same room three or four times in a row, or she might choose to enter different rooms. In all circumstances, the specter approached patients who, if awake, were instantly awash in cold. Shivering cold.

In 2012, Piedmont Newnan Hospital moved to a 136-bed facility on Poplar Road. The University of West Georgia acquired the Jackson Street hospital and grounds. The school recently began renovations on the old hospital.

But no one told the lady in white that the hospital was moving. She walks from room to room in the original building, twice daily at nine, checking for occupancy. Given the luxury of eternity, she'll still be at her rounds when the building has been fully remodeled.

Not everything a university scholar needs to know is in the school's guidebook. Students who find themselves in the renovated building at nine must learn to bring along a sweater and perhaps a pair of gloves. The lady in white will see to it.

SAVANNAH

Born into a wealthy and influential family in 1791, Mary Telfair bucked tradition and never married. She also enjoyed talking politics, which was frowned upon for women in the 1800s in the genteel South. When she died in 1875, Mary let her money speak for her. She bequeathed funds to establish a women's hospital in the port city. Opened in 1886, Telfair Hospital for Females was the first facility in Georgia created to provide medical care exclusively for women. Upon adding a nursing school in 1900,

Telfair Hospital established another first in Georgia.

Telfair Hospital served long and well at the corner of Drayton Street and Park Avenue, ultimately merging with Candler Hospital. In 1980, a new Candler facility was built and the original Telfair building was sold.

And that was when the ghost of Mary Telfair appeared. She has since been seen wandering from one end of the Victorian structure to the other, searching for her hospital.

Some helpful individual needs to tell Mary where to go. But word around town is that she has little patience with the men and women of modern Savannah and refuses to listen to them. Until a kindly ghost from a bygone era arrives from the afterlife to accomplish this communication, the ghost of Mary Telfair will likely linger.

WINDER

A ghost walks the old Barrow County Hospital building, now part of the expanded Barrow Regional Medical Center.

A former security guard was continually disturbed just before three o'clock each morning by strange sounds in a portion of the hospital used as offices. One night, the guard rode the elevator to the locked offices to satisfy his curiosity about what could possibly be going on up there. He met an individual in a hospital gown, and nothing else, strolling the hallways.

Nothing else includes the person's head, arms, legs, and body. The blue gown, clearly occupied, floated a foot or two above the floor.

KENTUCKY

END OF THE ROAD
WAVERLY HILLS SANATORIUM, 4400 PARALEE LANE, LOUISVILLE

IT ALL BEGAN INNOCENTLY enough and with the best of intentions.

Waverly Hills Sanatorium sits on land where a simple one-room schoolhouse was constructed in 1883. Because of her admiration of a series of Sir Walter Scott novels, the teacher, Lizzie Harris, named the school Waverly. It stuck. The rise of wooded land, now accessible at the end of Paralee Lane, is known as Waverly Hill.

Designed to accommodate approximately 40 patients, a simple two-story tuberculosis hospital was built at the location in 1910. Due to an epidemic of TB infections, it wasn't long before the hospital was overcrowded. Within a scant ten years, more than 140 patients were housed there.

A much larger and more impressive building was in place by 1926. Boasting space for at least four hundred patients, the new Waverly Hills Sanatorium was the best-equipped facility of the time. Four large gargoyles perched atop the Piedmont roof. Brick towers guarded the entrance. Stacked wings of windows spread to either side. An altogether colossal and intimidating building, Waverly Hills didn't quite look like a place where anyone would want to live. Or die. It most resembled a prison, or perhaps an appropriate place for a few dozen Dr. Frankensteins.

In the 1920s, a tuberculosis sanatorium was by definition a combination boardinghouse and hospital. Because TB was highly contagious, those known to be afflicted were not allowed to live among the general population. The infection typically and initially attacked the lungs and

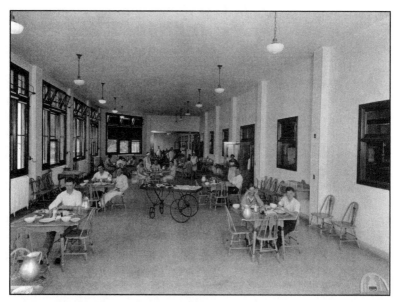

Patients at Waverly Hills in Louisville, Kentucky, 1926
CAUFIELD & SHOOK COLLECTION, UNIVERSITY OF LOUISVILLE PHOTOGRAPHIC ARCHIVES

was spread when people with active TB coughed. The classic symptom of tuberculosis is a chronic cough. Blood eventually appears with the cough, as does recurring fever, night sweats, and, as other vital organs are infected, dramatic weight loss. Chronic fatigue follows, often accompanied by deformity of the fingernails.

Tuberculosis has been around for some time. Researchers have located tubercular decay in the spines of Egyptian mummies dating from 3000 to 2400 B.C. Hippocrates identified phthisis in 460 A.D. as the most widespread disease of the time. Phthisis, likely a form of pulmonary tuberculosis, was said to involve fever and the coughing up of blood and was almost always fatal.

Folklore and superstition associated tuberculosis with vampires. When a person died of TB, other family members were often infected and would soon lose their health. People believed the resulting deaths were caused by the deceased's draining the life from his or her kin.

In 1815, one in four deaths in England was due to consumption, an early name for the affliction. The disease was named tuberculosis in 1839. It was also sometimes known as "the white plague."

One early treatment effort in Kentucky came in 1845, when Dr. John Croghan, the owner of Mammoth Cave, south of Louisville, brought a number of people with active tuberculosis into the cave to live. The good doctor hoped to cure the disease with exposure to a constant temperature and the purity of the cavern air. His patients died within a year.

Tuberculosis shortened life considerably. In the 1920s, most TB patients lived no longer than two years. Although widespread quarantines lessened the epidemic, that was little comfort for people with active tuberculosis, who were separated from their communities, families, and pets.

As at other TB institutions across America, patients at Waverly Hills lived in their own little world. Though not for long. Waverly Hills Sanatorium was the end of the road. Many experimental treatments and potential cures were attempted there. Some were brutally painful. A large number of patients who volunteered for experiments were left with horrific scars and bodily disfigurement. None got better.

In 1961, the discovery of an antibiotic that cured tuberculosis brought an end to TB hospitals. Quarantining was suddenly obsolete. Waverly Hills closed. Renovated, it served as a geriatric facility for several years. The building was vacated in 1980. Over the years, it lost many of its windows, and its interior was exposed to the elements. Before the structure fell into total ruin, it was purchased in 2001 by Charlie and Tina Mattingly. The undaunted couple is devoted to restoring the former hospital and sharing its history with visitors. They're doing a fine job of both.

It is estimated that as many as sixty-three thousand people died at Waverly Hills, which is often considered the most haunted place in the world. The owners prefer to describe the ominous structure and its grounds as "spiritually active."

Just outside Room 502, visitors have heard the creaking of a weight, as if it is being dangled from a rope. Walking through the room causes the weight to swing. Speculation is that a vivacious and popular nurse named Becky is still in the room. She was perhaps a little too vivacious. The unmarried nurse found out she was pregnant and was informed at about the same time that she had contracted tuberculosis. She hanged herself. Always on the move in life, Becky has found a way to keep swinging in the beyond.

Tunnels run beneath the former sanatorium. An entrance to the tunnels stands head-high in the woods like a stone bunker with a doorway. Visitors may, although it isn't advised, stroll into the opening. This is where ghosts are often heard. Upon entering the tunnels from this location, visitors may be met with the howls of the Waverly Hills dead. Hollow shadows that look like dark fog the size of people are known to appear as the howling intensifies. When the shadows disappear, footsteps run ahead in the tunnels. The rapidly retreating footfalls stop suddenly, as if waiting to be followed. Visitors who venture onward find that the sound of running soon returns, heading back toward the entrance. Then the footsteps stop again. Quickly, they turn around and advance at a rapid pace into the darkness. Ahead, a candle that is not there flickers, then dies. The sound of running entirely disappears. The howling abates. Someone coughs.

Visitors may go farther into the tunnels if they wish. Few do.

Besides, there are plenty of ghosts above the ground at Waverly. Visitors sometimes see the ghost of a child eager for playmates. Others catch sight of a ball bouncing along a hallway—a ball that disappears when it comes into contact with a wall. Full-body apparitions are common. One is a shaggy-looking man with frizzy hair.

Public tours of Waverly Hills are regularly scheduled. Though the old sanatorium is decidedly forbidding, the owners insist that not all of its ghosts are scary.

"We have a spirit here named Tim," Tina Mattingly says. "Sometimes, he puts off good vibes." She smiles rather wistfully, as if the phenomenon of a happy ghost fails to occur often enough at Waverly Hills.

Good vibes are appreciated at the end of any road. One certainly hopes that those who found earthly finality at the end of Paralee Lane think so.

TEAM SPIRIT
LEESTOWN DIVISION VA MEDICAL CENTER, 2250 LEESTOWN ROAD, LEXINGTON

ESTABLISHED IN 1931 by the newly created Veterans Administration, the Leestown Division VA Medical Center has always provided a wonderful setting for the recuperation of war veterans. As well as offering primary care, the institution excels at inpatient treatment for post-traumatic stress disorder. The Leestown VA also specializes in hospice and respite services for veterans, geriatric care, and therapy for mental-health and substance-abuse issues.

The original four-story brick hospital building, still in active service, was listed on the National Register of Historic Places in 2012. The facilities currently occupy more than 40 buildings on 135 acres. The campus includes plenty of trees and space for outdoor activities. Although some recovering veterans in years past worked the farm fields on the accompanying acreage, today's patients are more likely to be found taking advantage of the horseshoe pits, miniature golf course, and jogging trails. Much of the tree-covered, park-like campus is just right for an afternoon stroll—or roll, for those in wheelchairs.

Grayson Bruce found himself housed at the Leestown VA shortly after his service as a United States Army Ranger in the Vietnam War. The last thing he needed was noise. Mostly, he wanted to be left alone. There were many things he needed to stop remembering. Grayson had his own ghosts. He was haunted by war.

Grayson walked the campus daily, looking for places where he could be alone. He was also comfortable walking the woods in darkness.

It was pitch dark the night he was scared into a sudden and trembling sweat by a loud noise in the woods. It was a night without a moon. Grayson wandered the paths, ambling from one spot to the next. He thought about the things he had on his plate tomorrow. Another session with the doctor, who kept telling him they were a team, and one after that with a group.

During the last appointment, the doctor had spoken sternly. "You've wandered around the issues enough," he said. "It's time you hit it straight. Get on the bus with the rest of us or get out of here. Your life isn't baseless. It means something, and what it means to you is what you have to figure out."

"I don't know what you want from me," Grayson said.

"It's time you play ball," the doctor said. "Just run the bases. That's what I want from you. We're all here to back you up."

Not far from a road now called Opportunity Way, Grayson swiftly dropped to his belly in the sparse woods upon hearing a loud whack to his left. It sounded like a tree breaking in half. He feared he was hit. Brilliant light briefly flooded his vision.

He was safe, Grayson decided. Lying face down on the ground covered with a scattering of autumn leaves, he panted like a dog and struggled to remember something pleasant, something before Vietnam.

There was nothing before Vietnam, he concluded. Nothing that mattered.

That's when the former Ranger began to hear voices. A man called to someone in an open field edging the woods. Someone with a booming voice answered. They spoke in American English. Confident he was no longer in the Mekong Delta, Grayson rose to his hands and knees. Soon, he was standing up, able to swallow again, to breathe normally. He was also able to walk.

"How many times you going to call that one?" a bulky man asked.

The figure in the field wore a long-sleeved wool sweatshirt with striped pajamas for pants. No one was in front of him. No one was behind. The man was alone, as far as Grayson could see. And for some reason, Grayson could see him quite well—so well that it might have been daytime.

The stranger kept talking.

"Come on, come on," he said. "Get it to me."

Grayson approached, then nearly bolted when he heard a sudden slap. The crouching man came to his feet and swung his right hand forward like he was swatting a fly. He turned around and looked at Grayson.

"About time," he said. "Where have you been?"

Grayson motioned with a sideways move of his head. "Halfway around the world," he replied.

"Yeah, we all been there. I made it to Berlin." The man rubbed the side of his face with the back of his hand. "Why don't you take my place for a bit? I got to find the latrine."

Before the strange man in striped pajamas walked away, he held out his empty hand.

"Take this," he said.

The man moved his hand from his chin to the top of his head and tossed something toward Grayson. When Grayson looked down, a catcher's mask was at his feet. He picked it up and put it on. Suddenly, there was a leather mitt on his left hand, and he was wearing striped pajama bottoms and a long-sleeved wool sweatshirt.

They all were. A man carrying a baseball bat lifted it off his shoulder and scowled at Grayson, who dropped into a crouch behind home plate. Before the pitch came, he heard a voice behind him say, "Move your glove up when you catch the fastball or the ump won't call it a strike. He's blind as a bat."

"Save it for the dolls in France," the umpire growled in reply.

For the rest of the night, Grayson couldn't remember a thing about Vietnam.

What he remembered when he woke up was that he'd gotten on base twice. One of these nights, Grayson swore, he was going to touch home plate. But these guys were tough. It would take a couple weeks.

The Leestown VA has been the site of many strange occurrences over the years and is reported to be home to a number of ghosts. Phantom screams and moans are heard in the hallways. The sound of a door slamming shut when it is still open occurs in some patient rooms. Disembodied voices are heard talking and shouting at all hours, indoors and out. Strange lights move through the buildings.

Grayson Bruce is himself a ghost, having forgotten he'd committed suicide before taking a walk that night. People at Leestown Division VA Medical Center who keep their ears open while standing near the open field by Opportunity Way are likely to hear the sounds of Grayson and his teammates taking a second swing at life.

CRYING OUT LOUD
HAYSWOOD HOSPITAL,
WEST FOURTH AND MARKET STREETS,
MAYSVILLE

DOCTORS COMMONLY MADE HOUSE CALLS in the 1950s and for a few years beyond. At the same time, women across the South were comfortable having their babies at home. Jacki Treese, however, didn't have a doctor and didn't know a midwife.

Still single, and pregnant when she shouldn't have been, the young brown-eyed girl had only her father to turn to. He said that having a baby was the same thing as birthing a cow, except getting a baby out was easier. You cut the cord and slapped the baby till it cried. Then you washed it off some. He could handle it with the help of a little hot water and a couple of towels. He wouldn't name it, and neither would she.

In preparation, Mr. Treese had his daughter cut her hair short.

"You're going to sweat when it happens," he told her. "Long hair will just get in the way."

Jacki lived in seclusion in her father's house in Maysville, Kentucky, the Ohio River just a few blocks away. He preferred that no one in town, or anywhere else, know that his daughter was pregnant. Ever. He'd take the baby and sell it in secret. Or give it to the church at the edge of town. Jacki could leave afterward, if she wanted. Until then, the decisions were up to him. His daughter never made the right ones, after all. She was pregnant and barely fourteen.

If giving birth pained his daughter some, well, maybe it should. If it hurt enough, she wouldn't go out and do it again, he figured. Having a baby was no worse than having a tooth pulled. And you could do both at home.

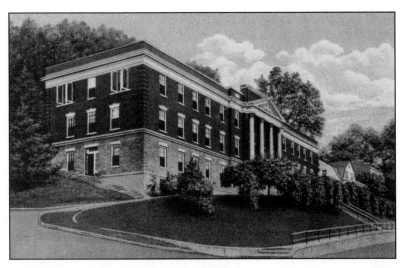

Hayswood Hospital in Maysville, Kentucky

In 1954, it rained most of August along the Ohio River. Jacki, as fat as a pumpkin, couldn't sleep one night. The weather was too loud. Her baby had been kicking up a storm the past two days. And now there was an actual storm. She sat by the window with the lights off and listened to the thunder. She believed the rumbling and the cracks of lightning meant the baby was ready to come out and be a person now.

She wondered if the baby, boy or girl, would be born with freckles the same as hers. She'd count them. Perhaps the newborn would look like its father, although she really couldn't imagine that.

Her dad slept through the thunder and lightning, the pounding rain. It wasn't her fault that no noise on earth would wake him once he started snoring.

Jacki put his hat on. She held her stomach with one hand and slipped out the door barefoot. A sizzle of lightning stabbed the sky. The street looked like a river.

She was a block from Hayswood Hospital when she realized something was wrong inside her. She leaned sharply forward, clutching her pumpkin stomach with both hands. Rain poured from the brim of her father's hat. Her dress was soaked through.

"Not now this minute," she said out loud. "Not now at all."

She couldn't stop yet. Jacki wanted her baby born on hospital sheets, not in sheets of rain.

Her feet were spread more widely than normal when she walked. Jacki's body wanted to sit down and scream. Instead, the girl about to be a mother willed her knees to hold them both up as she trudged on. She saw through the rain that the lights of the hospital were on. They always were, she knew. She'd been watching the place for months now. Three stories of lighted windows. Four white columns standing out front.

Her feet bathed in rain, Jacki stood on the street in front of the building and felt a new pain. It was a deep one that shot to the surface like a jagged bolt of lightning. The pain slammed her hard and burned like fire at the same time. She stood in the beams of headlights that approached and moved on as a car drove past her, sloshing through rainwater, its windows up.

Jacki realized she couldn't climb the steps up the little bit of hill in front of the hospital. She'd have to go around to the sloping drive. Like counting freckles one by one, she took a step and then another one. When she was partway up the slope, there was another brilliant stab of lightning and a deep roll of thunder. Blood and something else trickled down the inside of her legs. The rain mixed in, thinning it. *One more freckle*, she thought. *One more step.*

She had to stop counting when the pain hit her again. She couldn't help it. And she couldn't help her baby. It had stopped kicking and moving around inside her about two blocks ago. It was dead weight inside her stomach, and her body wanted rid of it. Just like her dad did.

She fell forward and stayed there while the rain washed away a profusion of new blood. Jacki felt like she was being cut open. She wanted to scream but couldn't. She managed to get herself to her hands and knees. She crawled forward, then collapsed again on her stomach. This time, she was dead. She'd meet her baby in heaven.

Because of the hat Jacki wore and her short hair, the nurse who saw her first thought she was a fat man who was drunk or had drowned.

"When the thunder stopped, I heard a baby crying outside," the nurse said. "We reached her as soon as we could."

It wasn't soon enough. And babies not born don't cry.

The rain slapped the ground as staff members carried Jacki into the hospital. The baby came out. They cut the cord and wrapped the bodies in clean sheets.

Her father wanted her buried with her baby. Since the child was still-born, he instructed the undertaker that one casket would do just fine.

"Nobody named that kid," he said. "No need to write it down."

A steady rain fell the day Jacki's casket was interred. Rain pelted the river as dirt was shoveled on top of her.

And every night it rained after that, people heard a baby crying outside Hayswood Hospital. A few said they saw a woman in a man's hat holding a baby in her arms.

Hayswood Hospital closed in 1983. The brick building stands empty today, waiting for a purpose. Its doors have been boarded over with sheets of plywood. Inside, much of the copper wiring has been taken, and the furniture is gone. Vandalism and trespassing have become regular occurrences. According to inspections conducted by the city, enough asbestos and lead paint are inside to make the expense of remodeling, or even demolition, entirely impractical.

Just outside the broken windows of the vacant rooms, a baby cries when it thunders or rains. It's been crying for sixty years. And for sixty years, Jacki, wearing a fedora soaked by rain, has rocked in her arms the baby that was never born. She softly, lovingly whispers its name. Cars slosh through the water on the street, their tires hissing. The Ohio River rolls on by.

OTHER KENTUCKY SIGHTINGS

ASHLAND

At the urging of the Franciscan Sisters of the Poor, Our Lady of Belle-fonte Hospital was created as a not-for-profit facility in 1956. Today, the expanded hospital is reported to be benignly haunted by the ghost of a former nurse known only as Fannie. The nurse enjoys briefly visiting patients in the middle of the day. Fannie is most often witnessed smiling in the doorways of patient rooms. Once seen, the grinning ghost goes away. But her smile is not forgotten. When nurses enter a room to find a patient smiling, they are apt to quip, "You must have seen Fannie."

Bellefonte Hospital currently enjoys the distinction of a five-star patient satisfaction rating from Professional Research Consultants, ranking it in the top 10 percent of hospitals in the United States.

BARDSTOWN

A two-story tavern built by Duncan McLean in 1812 originally housed the Bardstown post office and McLean's tavern downstairs. The upstairs rooms were rented to travelers. Now known as McLean House, the old tavern saw service as a hospital during the War Between the States. Over time, the ghosts of anguished soldiers have become permanent residents of the historic structure.

A local woman volunteered at the hospital to paint miniature watercolor portraits of dying soldiers, preserving their faces for family members. Her name is not recorded by history. The miniatures, too, are long gone, carried off by surviving soldiers or sent home with the bodies of less fortunate men.

Today, the painted faces, usually grim and determined, appear life-sized on the upstairs bedroom walls at night. Witnessing one is at first like seeing your own face in a mirror—only the face is not yours and there is no mirror. The faces quickly disappear when the lights are turned on.

Some believe the miniaturist created a wish among the dying to leave their full-sized faces behind in a permanent way.

CAMPBELLSVILLE

The building that now houses Campbellsville University's Gosser Fine Arts Center was previously Holy Rosary Hospital. Purchased in 1978 for use by the university, Holy Rosary had for more than two decades provided medical care to the surrounding population. Locals referred to it as a "birthing hospital," for good reason. Lots of Campbellsville babies were born there.

Providing ample space for recitals and other performances, Gosser currently houses the university's School of Music. Rehearsals in recent years have been attended by at least one appreciative, though unseen, newborn, who seems to prefer choral presentations. Instrumental rehearsals are often interrupted by the sound of a baby's crying, though no baby is present. The crying ceases when the rehearsal baton is tapped three or four times to regain the musicians' disrupted attention.

CORBIN

As many repurposed medical facilities prove, one doesn't have to visit a hospital to be haunted by a hospital.

An apartment building for senior citizens in Corbin, Kentucky, was built on the site of the recently demolished Memorial Hospital. The removal of a structure, however, rarely relocates the ghosts who live there. Some spooks prefer to stay.

The most recent manifestation in the new apartments is the recurring apparition of a tall man wearing a surgical mask, who is most often seen standing in front of the kitchen stoves of the homes he visits. He quickly vanishes when approached.

FORT CAMPBELL

Blanchfield Army Community Hospital, which provides health care for approximately one hundred thousand active-duty and retired soldiers and their families, has replaced the World War II–era hospital and morgue at Fort Campbell. Today, the two original brick buildings straddle the line between the living and the dead.

An enclosed walkway connects the buildings. This passage from hospital to morgue, from hope of life to certainty of being dead, is reported to be the most haunted location at Fort Campbell. Several servicemen wearing United States Army uniforms ranging from World War II tan khakis to the camouflage fatigues of the war in Afghanistan are seen walking the passage day and night.

"You don't really notice how they're dressed until they're close," said a soldier assigned to guard the old hospital at night. "And you don't notice that their eyes are blank until they're already past."

The soldier said he frequently calls out to the passing soldiers, but none of them pauses or replies.

HAZARD

The old UMW Miners Memorial Hospital in Hazard is now an office building and part of the University of Kentucky. Spirits remain active there. And one, at least, is quite vocal.

Those who wait long enough near the lobby entrance of the refurbished facility will hear a female voice loudly calling out a name. Minutes of silence pass. The name is called again. Finally, and much more quickly, the name is called a third time.

Those who have heard the ghost say that if you wait long enough, you'll hear the ghost call out a new name. Rumor is, when the name called out matches your own, you're dead.

LOUISVILLE

The original Women's Infirmary on South Sixth Street in Louisville was erected in 1892 to offer medical care to underprivileged women. It was eventually closed as a hospital and divided into apartments. The apartments are still occupied, by the living and at least a few of the dead.

At the turn of the twentieth century and for years afterward, a difficult birth more than occasionally resulted in the death of the mother. Many times, the newborn survived.

In 1946, a soldier home after World War II rented an apartment in the building, only to discover he wasn't alone. A tearful, pleading voice filled his living room day and night.

Being a religious man, the war-seasoned veteran called in a priest to bless the apartment. The voice changed into a mournful, unceasing moan in the presence of the priest, who quickly informed the tenant that more than a blessing was called for. The priest performed an exorcism, during which the apparition of a distraught woman appeared. She had a question for the priest.

When the ritual was over, the tenant returned. The priest told him that if he heard the female voice again, to tell her the baby was okay.

"Say he grew up and had a full life and that he is fine now," the priest said.

"I will," the veteran promised. "And I am."

PARIS

The abandoned tuberculosis sanatorium in Paris, Kentucky, was demolished in 2012. A ghost wearing a wedding gown, tiara, veil, and train was documented to have inhabited the grounds between the main hospital and the nurses' quarters while the facility was housing patients. It is said she still makes appearances, but only on nights of a full moon. Apparently, she intends to be seen. Always carrying a bouquet, she walks slowly to a given spot and stops. There, she throws the clutch of bridal flowers over her shoulder and disappears.

It has been suggested that someone's catching the bouquet before it hits the ground will rid the location of the ghost.

SMITHLAND

Smithland is an old town situated at the confluence of the Cumberland and Ohio rivers. Cumberland Marine Hospital, which once occupied a building on Mill Street, is thought by many to have been brought to use as a hospital during the War Between the States. That's not the case. State congressional records of both Ohio and Kentucky document a toll being charged in 1829 for commercial shipping on the Ohio River to support services at Cumberland Marine Hospital.

No one knows for sure how long the bearded face appeared in the window of Cumberland. The ghost face trapped in the glass was known to exist in the late 1800s. In fact, people traveled to Smithland for no other purpose than to gaze upon that face, said to resemble that of God. Lightning ultimately shattered the window.

Today, the marine hospital no longer exists. Locals are still cautious of the area. Few have the courage to tramp about the site. Superstition lives on in Smithland that anyone who steps on or otherwise disturbs even the smallest shattered sliver of the original window will be haunted by the bearded face's appearance in a window of their home.

VERSAILLES

The fourth floor of Bluegrass Community Hospital is haunted by a fourteen-year-old girl named Julie. She has a cast on her arm, and her head is bandaged as if from recent surgery. Julie's appearance is most often noticed by nurses after the mischievous ghost sets off the alarm light above the doors of unoccupied patient rooms.

LOUISIANA

GHOST IN A JAR
LA PHARMACIE FRANÇAISE,
514 CHARTRES STREET,
NEW ORLEANS

IT WAS 1859 when Catherine Simon, known simply as "Tuttie" when she was working as a dancer in the cabaret just blocks away, stood in front of the apothecary at 514 Chartres Street in New Orleans. She hesitated to go inside, but her dire need to resolve a problem soon overcame her reluctance.

She entered and spoke a few words. Following this brief consultation, the door was locked. A sign that the shop was temporarily closed was placed in the window. Dr. Joseph Dupas ushered Tuttie upstairs.

The country's first registered pharmacist, Dr. Dufilho, had established the business in 1823. The sister-in-law of Dr. Dupas, Celeste Pauline, subsequently purchased the apothecary and its contents from the founder. Only a few years before Tuttie's visit, Dr. Dupas had found himself the sole proprietor of La Pharmacie Française. He quickly acquired the reputation of having an effective treatment for anything a person might need fixed. Many of his potions and elixirs were available no other place in the world. They were his own concoctions, those of Dr. Dufilho, and a few special elixirs created by others in New Orleans.

The doctor-pharmacist also provided hands-on medical cures in the rooms upstairs, where Tuttie now found herself alone with him.

"I will not undress," she informed him as he closed the door behind her.

"No need," the doctor assured his patient. "But what I have for you

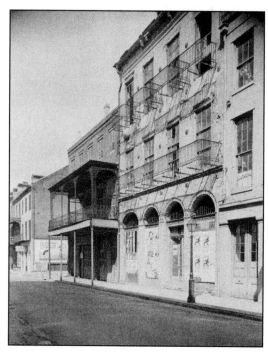

Chartres Street in New Orleans, Louisiana, outside La Pharmacie Française in the 1930s
LIBRARY OF CONGRESS, PRINTS & PHOTOGRAPHS DIVISION, LC-J7-LA-1032

cannot be shown to the public. I prefer you would consume the initial swallow while on the premises, so I might monitor your reactions and determine an appropriate dose."

"How much?"

"Three dollars," he said. "In gold, please."

As Tuttie opened her purse, the doctor retrieved a darkly colored bottle.

"Would the lady prefer a seat?" he inquired politely.

Tuttie placed three small coins on the corner of his desk.

"That I may remain standing is what I prefer," she said.

"As you wish, my dear."

He handed her a silver cup not much larger than a thimble. It was outfitted with a handle.

"It's a dosage spoon," the doctor said. "I invented it myself. It's deeper than a regular spoon and not as big around. When it is filled to the brim, we'll know exactly the amount you've consumed and the additional amount to be prescribed. You may take the spoon with you, if you wish, at no additional charge. I request only that it be carefully wiped clean after each use, and that you agree to return it to me when you are fully recovered."

"Will the cure take long?"

"Usually, within a week."

The doctor stepped to the window and, leaning into a bath of natural light, uncorked the bottle.

"Here," he said. He filled the dosage spoon and held it out for her. He otherwise did not move.

And neither did Tuttie.

"Here, in the light," the doctor said.

Once more for Tuttie, desire triumphed over hesitation, and she was soon standing between the doctor and a chair. The doctor smiled.

The medicine smelled like creosote and gin. "It stinks," she said, accepting the silver cup.

She held it to her lips and swallowed the potion. Her Creole eyes opened wide. The doctor wondered what she might be seeing.

Almost as quickly, her eyes closed. Tuttie dropped into the chair.

The doctor lifted her limp wrist and felt for a pulse. It was weak but there.

He held the apothecary bottle to Tuttie's mouth. Instead of pouring, he said, *"Entrer dans ma bouteille, mon cher. Avant de mourir."* Dr. Dupas squeezed her jaw with his other hand. "Into my jar," he urged. "Before you are dead. You will live forever if you come into my jar. *Tout de suite."*

He waited several moments before removing the open bottle from her lifeless face and replacing the cork. The doctor made a mental note to add an essential oil to the larger batch. Cherry, perhaps.

No longer detecting her pulse, he scraped the gold coins into his hand and left the room. He would return to empty her purse later. The doctor hurried downstairs. Her mouth now open as if to gasp air but wholly unable, Tuttie's lips slowly turned blue. Her tongue swelled with blisters.

Dr. Dupas patiently waited on other customers. Later, he returned to the upper floor. With great care, he sealed the corked top of the apothecary bottle with melted wax. He added a paper label with a simple notation in black ink.

He placed the sealed bottle—labeled *Tu'ti* because he was unsure how to spell her name—with the others on the top shelf of a mahogany cabinet he locked with a brass key attached to his watch chain.

Among his many recipes was one Dr. Dupas had learned through dedicated and focused experimentation, one he never entered in his pharmacopeia. It was his expert method of capturing a ghost in a thick, sticky elixir and sealing it inside a jar.

History has since confused Dr. Joseph Dupas with a near relative named James, who died in 1854. The pharmacist Joseph Dupas died in 1867 from advanced syphilis. Although he had created a number of concoctions to cure that ailment, including one that contained mercury, none proved an effective treatment for the doctor himself.

Records from the first half of the 1800s indicate that severe side effects accompanied the ingestion of mercury for syphilis, not the least of which was madness. Many did not survive the painful cure. One who did was the English poet Lord Byron, who was described by a contemporary as "mad, bad and dangerous to know." The same might be said of Dr. Dupas.

Now a museum, La Pharmacie Française is open to the public. The treatment rooms upstairs are known to be haunted by Dr. Dupas. It is believed he moves the items on display. People are also said to experience shortness of breath and pronounced discomfort when he is present. When asked, those who staff the museum will discuss the ghost of Dr. Dupas at length.

A fair number of ghosts as yet unmet also remain at La Pharmacie Française. They, like Catherine Simon, are sealed inside bottles on the top shelf of a locked cabinet.

CASKET GIRLS
URSULINE CONVENT HOSPITAL,
1100 CHARTRES STREET,
NEW ORLEANS

THE SISTERS OF URSULA, an order of French nuns devoted to service and the education of women, arrived in New Orleans in 1726, more than seven decades before the Louisiana Purchase. Among other acts of charity, the sisters provided medical care for victims of malaria and yellow fever. They were also quick to establish the Ursuline Academy for Girls upon their arrival. Instruction at the academy began in 1727.

The Ursuline Convent, housing a hospital, orphanage, and school, was completed in 1752. Noted for its famously shuttered windows, it still stands at the corner of Chartres Street and Ursulines Avenue. A rare survivor of eighteenth-century fires that destroyed most of the French Quarter, the convent is the sole intact building from the French colonial period in the United States. The wounds of both British and American soldiers were tended to in the same building during the Revolutionary War and the 1815 Battle of New Orleans.

Fanciful tales of the girls of Ursuline Academy account for the majority of vampire legends in New Orleans today. But there were no vampires at the academy. This mistaken notion was the result of early accounts that referred to the female students from France as "casket girls," a phrase that is often misunderstood. Such stories told of the young female immigrants arriving on wooden ships, each wearily carrying a casket in her arms. The caskets were said to have contained the undead. The girls carried the polished boxes to the convent and up the cypress stairway to the attic. The shuttered windows were opened at night. Bats flew from the windows to

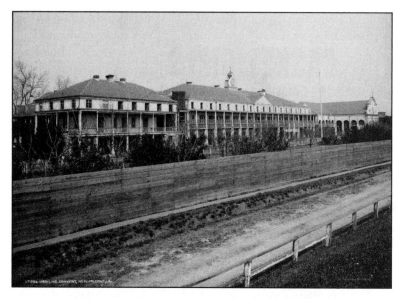

Part of the Ursuline Convent complex in New Orleans, circa 1910

the French Quarter for victims. Some amateur historians have even suggested that procuring a vampire from Europe was the cost of entry to the
school.

In truth, no blood was lost to vampires in New Orleans. The convent
is surely haunted, as are most buildings of its age, especially hospitals.
But no caskets were brought from France. The young women came to
New Orleans with the goal of marrying well. They provided services in
the hospital until being turned out as proper Catholic ladies to seek their
fates as wives and mothers in a new country.

The girls did not arrive with caskets. Most carried their worldly belongings in small carpet bags called *casquettes* in the Louisiana French of
the day. The expression referred to their poverty upon arrival.

What haunts the convent building today?

The shutters of the attic windows do fly open at night as the moon rises above the building. They shut again within the hour. Several of the impoverished French girls hoping to marry wealthy plantation owners succumbed to illnesses. It is said their ghosts return to check on the contents of their *casquettes*—their worldly goods and souvenirs from home. Casket girls received proper Catholic burials. Their travel bags and belongings, stored in the convent attic, were not buried with them. When the moon is high—either crescent or full—the shutters are pulled open from the outside so ghosts may enter to visit their past.

In 1824, the Sisters of Ursula moved from the convent to State Street. Today, ghost-free daytime tours of the Chartres Street convent and hospital, formal gardens, and church are provided on a regular schedule by docents. Named a National Historic Landmark in 1960, the convent currently houses a library and archives for the Archdiocese of New Orleans. Documents in the collection date to 1718.

The Ursuline Convent remains a popular stop during French Quarter ghost tours.

"We weren't too sure the ghosts would still be here," said a tour guide. "Many here believed the flood that came with Katrina might have washed the ghosts away. But we still have them in the attic at the old convent."

Ghosts are one more thing to be happy about in the French Quarter.

"Live people don't want to leave New Orleans, no matter the weather," the tour guide said. "And neither do the dead people."

STRAY CAT
ONE EYED JACKS,
615 TOULOUSE STREET,
NEW ORLEANS

DAVID PATTON DIDN'T LOVE stray cats at first, but he soon learned to.

He had a crush on a young lady who worked at the veterinary clinic on Toulouse Street. He watched her go to work in the morning and watched her leave in the evening. He would have followed her home, but he thought she wouldn't like that.

When he went in for the first time, unsure what to say, he found her holding a cat in her arms. She asked him if he needed anything in particular.

What he needed was to know her name.

"Oh, yes," he said. "Yes, I do. Uh . . ." David looked away from her questioning gaze.

"Yes?"

"Do you have any cats with curly hair?"

"We're a clinic for small animals," she said. "Not a pet store."

"I see."

"No big dogs," she added. "No dogs at all, really. Just birds and cats."

She stroked the mound of purring fur and peered at David. She was beautiful—so beautiful that David lost all confidence. He felt ragged. His hair wasn't trimmed. His shoes were scuffed.

"You need a job or something?"

David shook his head. Why would she think that? He started to tell her he taught piano at Miss Polly's but couldn't bring himself to say a word.

"Something to eat? I have a sandwich behind the counter. I can give you half."

She stared at him in a curious manner. She must have thought he was homeless. He had to say something.

"My name is David," he said. "What's yours?"

Cheryl said it to him, and he left.

David didn't go back for a couple weeks, but he watched when he could. People walked in the door with mostly cats.

The veterinary assistant was wearing a ruffled white blouse on the Thursday when David reentered the clinic. This time, he carried a yellow cat that had scratched his hand when he picked it up in an alley across the street. It had curly hair, which was why he had asked about cats with curly hair in the first place.

Her mouth was attractive when she talked. And triple that when she smiled.

Cheryl came around the counter. "What's the problem?"

"Fleas," David said. "And I think he needs a bath."

When she took the cat from him, their hands touched. She stepped through a curtained doorway behind the counter. When Cheryl returned, she gave him a form to fill out. He named the cat Dandy on the piece of paper. Once he finished with the form, she took it from him.

"We need a dollar down," she said.

David handed it to her.

"He's not yours, is he?" she asked.

"Not now," David said. When he smiled, she smiled back.

For the next several weeks, whenever he was able to catch a stray, he brought it to Cheryl. And once he brought a rose to give her for helping him. Over time, Cheryl grew fond of the man who rescued homeless cats.

David died when a scuffle broke out late one evening in front of a house of ill repute. He was looking for cats when two men tumbled into the street and knocked him over. One was holding a knife. He fell on top of David, and so did the knife. When the police asked, nobody could remember who it was who had a knife. They couldn't remember much at all.

A grave in the cemetery has the name of David Patton cut into the stone. But David wasn't there the day he was buried. He was back on Toulouse Street, carrying a cat from the afterlife. All anyone could see of either of them was a pair of cat's eyes floating waist-high above the sidewalk. The eyes eventually made their way to the veterinary clinic. One or two times a week for as long as she worked there, Cheryl opened the door to let them in, along with a rose from David.

By the end of the 1930s, the clinic was bankrupt. Cheryl found employment elsewhere. When the bank sold the building to new owners, they quickly reopened the clinic. But it wasn't the same. The clinic now occupied only the lobby. Customers were often advised that the clinic was completely full and were given the name of a nearby animal hospital.

The clinic served as a front for an illegal gambling and drinking establishment for the next several years. No one seemed to mind when cats' eyes appeared throughout the place. The owner called them "Dandy cats," though he couldn't say exactly why.

Today, the classic French Quarter building is merrily and quite legally occupied by a bar and alternative live music venue, One Eyed Jacks. The owners hired a photographer to take photos before renovations. The resulting pictures included a large number of strange glowing lights the size of cats' eyes. Paranormal investigators spent several nights at the location and reported that the room filled with the smell of roses at night. The message "She misses him" was conveyed by a participating clairvoyant.

Customers and staff see the floating eyes, usually behind the bar near the front of the club. The "Dandy cats" don't mind the music or the crowds. It's where they live now.

And thanks to the dedication of the ghost of David Patton, another pair of eyes arrives once or twice a week, accompanied by the lingering scent of a freshly cut rose.

They say that night has a thousand eyes. On Toulouse Street in New Orleans, those eyes belong to cats.

OTHER LOUISIANA SIGHTINGS

BATON ROUGE

For those who need to cool off in Louisiana in the summer, Baton Rouge has just the place. Originally Baton Rouge General Hospital, the Guaranty Income Life and Broadcasting building is haunted by a ghostly touch of cold air. Employees report that the entire building is occupied by wandering ice-cold ghosts. The bottom floor, once the hospital morgue and now the cafeteria, is the coldest. Occasionally, people talk about experiencing a ghost when being surrounded by, or walking through, a cold spot. Employees attest that the ghosts don't fool around with a temperature drop of a degree or two. The manifestations are frigidly cold.

Drop by the offices someday. You may find employees chattering on about the ghosts.

GREENWELL SPRINGS

Greenwell Springs Mental Hospital recently closed. But not all the patients treated there are gone.

Louisiana's "Skunk Ape" is believed by many to be the ghost of a hairy giant housed for study at the hospital in the 1960s. He escaped his restraints and left the hospital to live in the woods along Greenwell Springs Road, where he survived by eating small forest creatures. Unwashed and smelly, the giant avoided contact with other people and died of a combination of exposure and old age. His rotted corpse was discovered by a hunting dog.

The giant's remains were buried in a pauper's grave and archived in the county records by a number, instead of a name. Those who tended to his burial noted that his hair was exceedingly thick and matted and covered the giant's entire body.

Today, the ghost of the Skunk Ape is seen in the headlights of cars traveling the winding Greenwell Springs Road. A powerful odor, noticed most when car windows are down, accompanies the sightings.

KEACHI

Not much remains of Keachi Women's College except ghosts. Although local historic buildings have been moved to the former campus, the college's original two-story building no longer exists. The town, despite having a population under 350, is home to 11 structures listed on the National Register of Historic Places.

The women's college initially served as a Confederate depot for medical supplies shipped overland from Mexico. During the Battle of Mansfield on April 8, 1864, and for some weeks afterward, it became an emergency Confederate hospital; the morgue was on the second floor. An estimated one thousand Confederates died in the battle.

Over time, Keachi has been alternately spelled as Keachie and Keatchie. But the ghosts don't care. The Keachi Women's College hospital grounds are their home, and they mean to protect it. The remains of a hundred Southern soldiers are buried in the Keachi Confederate Cemetery. Among them is a ghost in the distinctive uniform of the Keachi Highlanders, who guards the town by walking the roofs of buildings at the college. The Highlanders wore Scottish caps complete with side feathers and plaid kilts into battle, accompanied by two company bagpipers.

The skirted sentinel ghost is seen but not heard. Perhaps he chooses to remain silent in memory of his fallen brethren. Or perhaps he was permanently deafened before death by the clamor of battle, the roar of cannon fire, or a head wound.

He carries his loaded musket and fires it from the rooftops of the buildings. Some suggest the flash of his musket is intended to alert the town to the presence of Union forces. Others claim he fires his weapon as a locating signal for injured Confederates in need of medical attention. The flash of fire from a black-powder musket is seen several times each evening when the ghost is active, as occurs especially in April. The firing of the silent musket is considered by locals to be a harbinger of spring.

MONROE

Hospital beds can be haunted, too.

Ghosts became active in the 1895 Roland M. Filhiol house on Stone

Avenue in Monroe, Louisiana, when a hospital bed in a second-story bedroom was moved.

"Boy, was that a mistake," the owner said.

One ghost, named Larry by the owners, is believed to have been a tenant of the house at a time when it was divided into apartments. Larry died in his seventies, apparently in the bed, and he means to stay. He prefers that silence be maintained in the hallway outside his room.

A second ghost is that of a young girl, likely a relative of Larry's, who entertains the current house dogs by daily running the stairs. "The dogs aren't yet insane," one of the owners said, "but she's driving us bananas."

The latest report from Monroe is that Larry and the little girl bother the dogs when any piece of furniture is moved. Ghosts prefer things to stay as they were—especially when it's the bed they died in.

NEW ORLEANS

Located on Chartres Street one block from the old Ursuline Convent, Hotel Provincial occupies five buildings and is listed on the National Register of Historic Places. In 1722, the French military used the original site as a hospital. During the War Between the States, a Confederate hospital provided care at this location.

Building 5 of the current hotel complex, constructed on the site of the hospital, is considered the most haunted at Hotel Provincial. The building's ghosts are oblivious to being observed. Guests have opened the doors to their rooms to see a bandaged and bloody soldier writhing in pain on the bed, accompanied by audible moaning. The specters rapidly fade and are said to completely vanish by the time the lights in the room are turned on.

PINEVILLE

Central Louisiana State Mental Hospital opened in Pineville, just across the Red River from Alexandria, in 1906. A dairy barn and a cemetery were among the earliest facilities at the hospital. It is estimated that nearly three thousand former patients are interred here.

Many of the buildings on the forty-acre grounds are no longer in use.

Nestled among the trees on the campus is the original 1917 limestone and concrete building that saw many years of service as the hospital's morgue and pathology lab. In 1922 alone, fifty-six autopsies were undertaken inside the structure.

Now a museum, the handsome two-story Italianate Renaissance Revival building is known as Rose Cottage. The rather simple interior consists of two rooms on the ground floor and one large room above. But having one's body parts dissected and examined between death and burial is not so simple. That's where the ghosts come in.

Originating as bits of mist that collect nightly in the cemetery, the ghosts become fully visible—right down to the bootlace autopsy stitching on their chests and abdomens—as they make their way back, on hands and knees, from the cemetery to Rose Cottage. Apparently, they seek to be made whole again so they may rest in peace in their graves.

RUSTON

In the late 1970s, the old Ruston Hospital building on the south side of Hergot Avenue was donated to Louisiana Tech University. Now a facility for biomedical engineering, the twenty-three-thousand-square-foot brick structure is haunted by a ghost with an acute sense of smell and a lousy sense of direction. Known to operate the elevator in a most willy-nilly fashion, the ghost always manages to open the door to the empty elevator for anyone carrying donuts from nearby In-and-Out Donuts. Researchers in the building say the quickest way to get around inside is to bring a donut with you.

SLIDELL

Reggie, a former patient at Ochsner Medical Center–North Shore in Slidell, is another hospital ghost who likes to operate the elevator. Reggie has a fondness for women, especially nurses, to whom he has been known to introduce himself before fading into thin air. He also has a friend in the afterlife he sometimes brings with him. Too shy to make himself known, this ghost without a name appears as a dark mist that rapidly evaporates when the elevator door opens.

THIBODAUX

Ellender Hall, a six-story coeducational dormitory on the campus of Nicholls State University, is known for scratches on its interior walls. Constructed on the site of a Confederate hospital, the building appears to have trapped a former patient who died there during the War Between the States. A lost soul from the Confederate hospital is attempting to find his way home using a broken cavalry saber. But the door to the outside of the hospital is no longer where it used to be, so the ghost is cutting a new one. Even though he has managed only to scratch the walls thus far in his effort to create appropriate egress, the hacking ghost hasn't given up his goal.

The school song at Nicholls, "All Hail to Thee," includes the lines, "The echo of thy spirit rises, and fills devotion's cloudless sky. To thee we pledge our loyalty through all the years that are to be."

That's a lot of years for the abandoned and now trapped Confederate volunteer to continue to scratch the walls with his broken sword. But he seems dedicated to the task of using his weapon to make his way out of the building.

MISSISSIPPI

LOVE'S LAST LEG
WHITE ARCHES,
122 SOUTH SEVENTH AVENUE,
COLUMBUS

MARY OLIVER UNEXPECTEDLY attended the gathering at White Arches. It was a formal party held on the eve of the departure of Mississippi volunteers under the command of Jeptha Vining Harris. In May 1863, the local militia, organized by Harris, was ordered to leave Columbus to defend the riverfront at the besieged Confederate city of Vicksburg.

Citizens knew firsthand the cost of war. Following the Battle of Shiloh a year earlier, Columbus had become a hospital town. Maimed and wounded soldiers were sent to the stronghold on the Tombigbee River by train. Just about every large house in Columbus served as a hospital late in the war. Thousands of soldiers were buried in Friendship Cemetery on South Fourth Street.

As Union troops fought their way deep into Dixie, Mary found it peculiar to be attending a party. The gala was held in General Harris's lavish seventy-five-hundred-square-foot home, White Arches, on the banks of the Tombigbee. The chandeliers were lit in every room of the mansion, located just three blocks north of the cemetery. Guests were welcome to tour the home while a band played stirring tunes in the grand hall on the first floor.

Wearing her finest, yet ultimately plain, dress, Mary stood out from the superior and discriminating damsels of Columbus. She owned no jewelry. Not a single piece of lace. She stood out even more because she was unaccompanied by an escort. As far as the guests were aware, she had no personal connection to any of the uniformed soldiers leaving for Vicksburg the next day. Not even a private or a bugler.

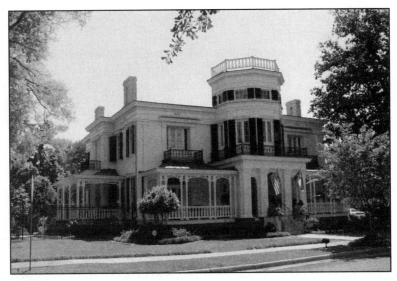

White Arches in Columbus, Mississippi
JEFFREY REED

Her association with one dashing officer of the Confederate militia was indeed private. The man secretly allied to Mary was Captain Edward Poteet, whose likeness had recently been published in the newspaper. The cause of her secret attachment was itself no secret at all. Poteet was married.

Mary lived alone in a small unpainted house inherited from her father. It stood near the little church far out Nash Road. No one knew who came and went at Mary's house.

Desperately in love, Mary attended the party, where she did not so much as cast a glance in the direction of Poteet. Total discretion was an expected habit among young ladies of the South.

Mary kept to herself at the party and quietly left. She departed so quietly, in fact, that some at the gathering thought she might have jumped from the tower roof of White Arches. The rumor persists to this day. In truth, Mary walked away after spending a few minutes wandering the house in misery. And misery followed her after the long walk home that evening in spring.

As the first wounded from Vicksburg arrived in Columbus, Mary volunteered at the busiest hospital, where she bandaged injured limbs and amputations. Only days later, Captain Poteet arrived in the back of a wagon, drawn swiftly from the train depot to a sudden stop in front of the hospital. He had been treated at a battlefield hospital and was deemed to have survived his injury but was not ambulatory. A musket ball had been cut from his leg, and he had a bandaged shoulder. The shattered bone just above the captain's knee was splinted into place as well as the Confederate surgeon could manage. Once he improved, Poteet would walk with a crutch, if he walked at all.

Poteet did not improve. Gangrene set in. The surgeon in Columbus cut away the increasing mass of dead flesh, but the hoped-for cure did not materialize. The leg was amputated just below the hip in an effort to stop the progress of the infection. Sadly, Poteet did not survive the surgery.

Mary was on the lawn of the hospital when the staff brought out the body of the man she loved. In the face of death, discretion was tossed to the wind. She rushed inside the hospital, where she located Poteet's severed leg. Mary wrapped it inside the white apron that fronted her floor-length dress and hurried away, clutching the piece of her lover in her arms.

The leg was all she possessed of him. Mary intended to keep that portion of her lover with her forever. He would become a part of her. And at the end of her life, they would be buried together for eternity.

As the moon lifted over the river, Mary turned her father's small house into a home hospital. By lamplight, she tenderly bathed her lover's leg. It was enough of him, she thought. It was all of him she had.

She removed her dress. Physical pain did not matter if it cured the anguish of a broken heart. Mary sewed his leg to her thigh one stitch at a time. Blood from repeated punctures through living flesh ran in soothing rivers down her leg—and his. She sewed deeply into her flesh to join his leg securely to hers. Now, it was Mary's body—not that other woman's—that nourished her lover.

She dressed before daylight and walked to the little church. But on this walk, she was accompanied. Mary was no longer alone in this life. She wondered that she might be insane. If that was the case, so be it. After spending time in the chapel, looking upon the cross of suffering and Christ's bloody crown of thorns, Mary began the three-legged walk to town. Others occasionally passed her. A woman in a carriage stared at Mary as if in shock. The man with her shouted to hurry the horse. Mary was dizzied by then—dizzied, she believed, by an accomplishment of love.

She sat beside the road and changed her mind. She didn't need Columbus. Mary stood. She was crying as she staggered along Nash Road. She swayed. She collapsed. She got up again and forced herself to hurry, to carry on. Leaving a trail of fresh blood, Mary died hobbling across a small bridge near the little church. She'd bled to death, her heart drained of all but love.

By the time Mary was buried in the churchyard, Poteet's leg had been removed and discarded as waste. Their bodily congress ended, Mary was disconsolate. She chose to remain on earth as a ghost rather than enter the afterlife without the touch of her one, true love.

Today, the ghost of the three-legged woman is often seen on Nash Road. Attracted to love, she appears outside cars parked for privacy late at night on turnoffs along the country lane. The three-legged woman is said to give cars a kick, then race them to the bridge.

Teens around Columbus know her best. They say if Mary gets to the bridge before you do, she'll stand in the middle of Nash Road and wait. It becomes a game of chicken then. And Mary isn't chicken. No matter how fast you drive, the three-legged ghost will kick your car from the bridge and into the creek.

White Arches is listed on the National Register of Historic Places. A brass sign notes the home's eclectic architecture and central three-story tower.

No sign has been placed on Nash Road regarding Mary Oliver or her three legs. The road she travels is gravel. The little church is gone.

HOME TO STAY
DUFF GREEN MANSION,
1114 FIRST EAST STREET,
VICKSBURG

FOLLOWING TWO MAJOR ASSAULTS by Union troops, Vicksburg came under siege in early summer 1863. Under the command of John C. Pemberton, who had lost three-quarters of his army in the two battles, the Confederates, with no reinforcements and dwindling supplies, gallantly held out behind heavy fortifications for more that forty days before surrendering the Mississippi stronghold on July 4.

Along with the Confederate defeat at the Battle of Gettysburg the previous day, the surrender of Vicksburg is considered by many historians to have been the turning point in the War Between the States. Among Confederates at Vicksburg, death was three times more common than survival.

Just as the battles and ultimate siege of Vicksburg had a major impact on the armies of the South, the lives of the citizens of the community were devastated. Even the wealthy among them were not spared from heartbreak, hardship, and tragedy.

Intending it as a wedding gift for his young bride, the former Mary Lake, Duff Green built a mansion in 1856 on a rise a short walk from the Mississippi River. By all accounts, Mary Green loved the place. Her children would be born and raised there.

Mary was advanced in pregnancy with her second child in May 1863. Her home was hit five times by Union cannon fire. Well aware of the need to save her house and to provide care for those falling around her, she hoisted a yellow flag, signaling that the mansion was being used as a

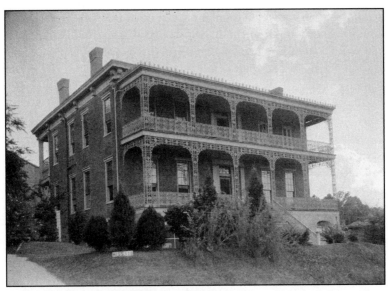

The Duff Green Mansion in Vicksburg, Mississippi
LIBRARY OF CONGRESS, PRINTS & PHOTOGRAPHS DIVISION, MISS,75-VICK,8-1

hospital. By custom of war, the mansion was no longer to come under fire.

Although she and her three-year-old daughter, Anne, were now relatively secure, the inside of the mansion quickly became a place of misery as the maimed and dying were treated. To provide more room for the surgeons and wounded soldiers, and perhaps to escape the moans and screams, Mary, Anne, and attending members of the household retreated to caves on the property. In one such shelter, while listening to the roar of cannons across the river, she gave birth to a son. She named him William Siege Green.

Mary anticipated regaining her cherished home upon the surrender of Vicksburg. She'd scrub the place from rafters to floorboards and tend her infant son. She would assist others ravaged by the misfortune of war. She'd see to it that her children learned the importance of peace and progress.

However, instead of regaining control of hearth and home, Mary found her mansion put to continuing service as a hospital. Both Union and Confederate troops in need of medical care moved in and out of the mansion. Surgeons and their assistants worked in shifts. Mary was not allowed to return.

The Duff Green Mansion was formally leased by the United States government later that year as a hospital for recuperating soldiers. And so it remained until 1866, when the estate was finally returned to its rightful owners.

Duff Green died in 1880. History does not record the date of the death of Mary Lake Green.

Perhaps that doesn't matter, since Mary still occupies the home she cherished. Her ghostly apparition walks from room to room in the restored mansion. No corner is off limits to her presence. And Mary is not alone. Her daughter, Anne, is with her, locked in time as a six-year-old, the girl's age when the Greens were allowed to come home after the war.

A couple visiting the mansion not long ago was perplexed when their young son made motions like he was throwing and catching something that wasn't there. When asked by his father what he was doing, the little boy replied, "I'm throwing the ball to Annie."

The mansion was purchased and fully restored in 1985. The new owners reportedly removed twenty-seven layers of paint.

Today, cannonball damage to the ceiling beams at the Duff Green Mansion remains as clearly visible as the apparition of Mary, who, daughter in hand, walks the grand staircase in the ballroom at precisely six o'clock, coming downstairs for dinner.

RATTLING RAT TEETH
HALLER NUTT MANSION,
140 LOWER WOODVILLE ROAD,
NATCHEZ

THE GHOSTS ARE AROUND BACK at Longwood, the not-quite-finished Haller Nutt Mansion in Natchez, Mississippi. Besides the fact that the upper two floors were never completed, Longwood is known for its octagonal shape, byzantine onionskin dome atop a central tower, and white-eyed ghost wearing a necklace of rattling rat teeth.

The house, a National Historic Landmark designed by architect Samuel Sloan, is considered a last burst of Southern opulence prior to the War Between the States. Cotton baron Haller Nutt commissioned the lavish edifice in 1859. Construction—featuring slave-made bricks—began early the next year. The war brought an end to construction in 1861, but not before the exterior walls were up and the first floor had been framed into rooms.

Nutt owned several plantations during his life and possessed considerable wealth. In 1860, he owned forty-three thousand acres and eight hundred slaves. Longwood was to be the master's house at Laurel Hill Plantation, the home to hundreds of slaves just outside Natchez. Perched on a bluff above the Mississippi River, Natchez had long been a center of commerce. It was perfect to have a large plantation nearby.

At the outbreak of war, Nutt, his wife, Julia, and their eight children moved into the unfinished octagonal mansion. While battles were being fought elsewhere, Nutt hurried his slaves to finish the interior. Those slaves lived in hastily constructed shanties directly behind the mansion. With them was a cook known only as Hettie. She boiled a variety of things in her cast-iron pots to feed the men working on Nutt's house. One of those things was rats.

Famed among the slave population in Mississippi for her potions and poultices, Hettie was a doctor of sorts for her displaced and wearied community. Word of her healing prowess spread throughout the Natchez area. Poor white men and women who could not afford a doctor visited the cook's shanty at night. They brought food to exchange for Hettie's curious potions, charms, and chants. Meat was a favored trade for treatment. A chicken, if one were available. If not, a dead possum would do.

It was said of Hettie that she could raise the dead.

As the war came to Mississippi, Natchez remained largely unscathed. Two civilians—an elderly man and an eight-year-old girl—died when a Union ironclad shelled the town from the river. The girl was hit by a shell fragment. The man succumbed to a heart attack. Union troops under Ulysses S. Grant occupied Natchez in 1863.

On a June night in 1864, a poor man walked to Hettie's shanty for help with a sore on his leg that would not heal. It was a busy night for Hettie. Slaves had been lashed that day for working too slowly on the second floor of the Nutt house and because two boards were missing from the lumber stacked outside. She looked at the man's leg, and then his eyes, and told him to return with alcohol, white paint, and a dead rat, if he could find one.

"And something to eat, for sure," she said.

Two days later, he complied. He left the chicken with its feathers on, in case she needed them.

The white man was soaked in sweat, which Hettie took as a good sign.

"The devil is in you," she said. "You're all a-sweat because the devil won't come out."

"The devil, you say?" the man asked, to be certain he'd heard correctly.

"Yes, sir, the devil is locked inside, sure. And he burns something awful when he gets inside a man. But don't you worry. We'll make him come out."

Pouring whiskey and white paint into the open sore on his leg certainly seemed to do the trick. The man yelped, swore, and danced around.

"Stop your cursing," Hettie told him. "It don't mean nothing to Satan. Now, sit back down and let me finish with you."

Two black men held him down. Hettie cut his leg with a knife and poured in more whiskey, more paint. The man nearly threw up from the pain.

"The devil likes whiskey," Hettie said. "But he don't like paint."

Hettie painted white circles around the man's eyes. The sweat was lifting. She tied a cloth bandage around his calf, over the wound. She tied a matching bandage on his other leg for balance.

"You're doing better already," she said.

She put her large face directly above the man's and looked into his eyes. He looked into hers.

"Now," Hettie said, "you're going to do as I say."

The black woman pulled the boiled rat from the pot and removed its jaw. She fashioned an amulet of the bone and its accompanying teeth by tying it with twine to a jute strap already strung with dried seedpods. She placed it around her patient's neck and tied it in back.

"You're cured now, sure," she said. "But you have a favor to complete. You go to the big brick house and walk inside the back door and ask for Master Nutt, then put some of your whiskey in your mouth. When he comes to see who you are, blow that whiskey in his face. You hear?"

Hettie had him eye to eye. The man nodded agreement.

"Then you're done and finished with it all. You can come back here and lay down for a spell."

Once he left, Hettie told the two slaves who'd helped her that she'd seen the devil in that man. When she'd looked into the man's eyes, the devil stared back.

"I got the old devil right where I want him. He's going to help us now, sure."

His trousers pushed up to his knees, his eyes circled in white paint, the man walked to the mansion, the seedpods around his neck rattling with every step. The pain in his leg had disappeared, he noticed. And he could see in the dark. Both these things surprised and pleased him.

When he reached the back door, he knocked. Haller Nutt told him to come inside and, somewhat flummoxed, asked why in the dickens the man was dressed like that.

"Somebody at the lodge get hold of you?" the plantation owner asked. "Is this your initiation?"

The man with a jaw of rat teeth tied around his neck didn't answer. Instead, he took a mouthful of whiskey from the bottle he'd brought with him and blew it in the plantation owner's face.

Nutt sputtered and coughed. He pushed the anonymous intruder from his home.

The man walked directly back to Hettie's shanty, where he lay down on a straw pallet—and was dead by morning. Hettie had known he was about to die by the black streaks up his leg from the open sore. There was nothing poor Hettie could do to cut the devil out of a white man.

Haller Nutt started coughing that night and couldn't stop. The doctor from Natchez came and went. Nutt died of summer pneumonia on June 15, 1864. He was buried in the Longwood cemetery, laid to eternal rest not far from the woods where a few days earlier slaves had buried a man wearing a jaw of rat teeth around his neck while Hettie sang songs to keep the devil in the ground.

The ghost seen today near Longwood is said to have white eyes and to walk like a zombie toward the octagonal house. Those who encounter him say he rattles when he walks.

To this day, an unmarked "coffin hollow" on the grounds causes the leaves in the trees to rattle when it is stepped on. Or so it seems.

The Nutt family continued living at Longwood after Haller's death. Julia was left with the responsibility of raising and educating several children during Reconstruction. She was said to always be kind to former slaves. She employed several, including a woman named Hettie, who served as the family's live-in nanny.

Longwood survived decades of neglect. Now one of Natchez's most popular attractions, though its upper floors are still unfinished, it is owned and operated as a historic house museum by the Pilgrimage Garden Club. In 2010, the mansion was used in the HBO series *True Blood* for the external shots of the fictional mansion of Russell Edgington.

OTHER MISSISSIPPI SIGHTINGS

BILOXI

The former Biloxi Regional Hospital on Bayview Avenue closed in 1986. The remodeled building now houses the Department of Marine Services for the Gulf of Mexico and the Mississippi coast.

When the hospital was active, dying patients would see two young girls standing by their beds. One was about five years old, the other a year or two older, according to nurses who worked at the hospital. A nurse who relocated to the new medical center on Reynoir Street recently stated that the two girls have yet to appear to any of the patients there.

Recent reports from the Department of Marine Services, however, indicate that the ghosts of two little girls are in the old building. They're rarely seen, but when they are, it's on the occasion of a permit or license being issued to someone who is going to die on his next boat trip.

DURANT

Castalian Springs, a popular health spa prior to the War Between the States, is now noted for its Confederate cemetery. In 1970, a Mississippi state historical marker was erected three miles east of a local structure that served as a boarding school for girls in 1854. The school was subsequently converted to a Confederate hospital, where wounded soldiers from the Battle of Shiloh were treated. The bodies of forty-three soldiers were buried along the dirt road.

Most recently, the clapboard structure has been used as a girls' summer camp. A tall, uniformed officer appears at the camp whenever someone sees a snake. Wearing a gray Confederate cavalry hat complete with gold cord, the duty-bound officer chases the snake away. Then he vanishes with a gentlemanly nod.

The war may be over, but in Castalian Springs, a soldier's job is never complete.

PORT GIBSON

On April 30, 1863, Confederate general Martin E. Green posted his brigade near Magnolia Church. Two forward sentries were assigned to the home of A. K. Shaifer, constructed in 1820. Believing nothing of consequence would occur until morning, the sentries were lax in their duties and fell asleep. Shortly after midnight, the house came under musket fire. One of the soldiers escaped the assault. The other died. Union general John A. McClernand then used the house as a hospital, where his surgeons tended troops wounded during the ensuing Battle of Port Gibson.

The house was donated to the state in the late 1970s. It came complete with battle scars from Minié balls and the ghost of the first Confederate casualty, the sentry caught by surprise in the Shaifer home. The Confederate ghost is an auditory one, known to shout shortly after midnight. The shout begins as a cry of surprise, followed by a low moan. Then a body can be heard falling onto the hardwood floor.

SARDIS

Sometimes, patients in pain must be temporarily restrained to receive triage and treatment, especially in emergency rooms. A beefy nurse who once worked at the old North Panola County Hospital in Sardis, Mississippi, was especially talented at restraint. According to recent reports, she still is, although she's dead. The hospital is long abandoned, so patients are few. The only way to enter is by trespassing, which is certainly not recommended. A stout ghost is known to grab anyone who ventures inside the closed emergency room and not let go.

UNION

Boler's Stagecoach Inn was once used as a field hospital and headquarters by Union general William T. Sherman, a man known as a pyromaniac and arsonist throughout much of the South.

Sherman, it is claimed by historians, did not burn the city of Union, Mississippi, because of its name. Nor did he torch Boler's inn.

The long, two-story clapboard inn has undergone extensive restoration of late. That has not, however, dislodged the ghost of a Union soldier who lives inside the building by day and guards the grounds at night. He is believed to be a paymaster of Sherman's army, who, through a mix-up of scheduling, arrived with a lockbox of gold coins after the general and his men had left the inn to continue their incendiary march through Mississippi. Fearful of being robbed, the soldier is said to have buried or otherwise safely hidden the cache. Left alone on the property for several days, he was "accidentally" shot by locals, who mistook him for a rabbit or a deer in the morning mist. His body was hastily buried so their mistake wouldn't be discovered. Many are convinced his ghost continues to haunt the location because the gold he is guarding has yet to be found.

VICKSBURG

Anchuca Mansion was used as an emergency hospital during the 1863 siege of Vicksburg. A young woman who volunteered as a nurse there was so frightened that she refused to venture outside the building during the siege.

Her ghost appears to relive her terror. She's back inside the house and still won't leave. The new owners of the mansion, now operated as an inn, report several other ghosts inside its walls as well.

VICKSBURG

Cedar Grove Hall, a Roman Revival mansion on the bluff overlooking the Yazoo River at its confluence with the Mississippi, was built for John Alexander Klein and his family in 1852. An attack from Union warships on the Yazoo in 1863 left a cannonball embedded in the wall of the parlor. Following the surrender of the city to Federal troops, the mansion was converted to a Union hospital, as were most large homes in Vicksburg.

Now a fancy inn and restaurant, Cedar Grove is haunted by the ghostly dual apparitions of a blinded and bandaged soldier in blue being led by the hand by a young girl in a striped dress. Together, the ghosts walk from Oak Street to the mansion's front steps. The girl is believed to be one of the children of John and Elizabeth Day Klein, the original own-ers of the home.

History has paid far too little attention to the plight of children whose families, homes, and cities have fallen prey to the devastation of war. Vicksburg would be the perfect place for further research.

VICKSBURG

Closed in 1989, Kuhn Memorial State Hospital sits abandoned and fallen into ruin. Mississippi's "urban spelunkers" often explore the tile halls of the first floor. But only those who venture to the upper floors have seen the ghosts who live there.

Kuhn was previously known as State Charity Hospital. Sixteen doctors and six Sisters of Mercy died in the facility while treating victims of a yellow-fever epidemic that ravaged Vicksburg in 1878. The ghosts are apparitions of those special victims, doctors and nurses who refuse to leave their patients in need of comfort and care. Sadly, the patients are no longer there.

Locally known as "the thirsty ghosts of Kuhn," the apparitions appear as though in pantomime. They beg for water and point to locations where patient beds once stood. Without making a sound, the ghosts vanish as quickly as they appear.

VICKSBURG

A multistory facade of blue tile and a cross identify the old Mercy Hospital, which occupies a hill a full forty feet above Grove Street. When it opened in 1957, Marcy was a state-of-the-art medical facility bustling with activity. But the hospital is now closed and silent, encircled by a tall chain-link fence topped by loops of razor wire. Its door securely locked, the facility has become a prison to the spirits of patients who died there and decided not to leave while they had the chance. Ghosts are seen at night pushing against the chain-link fence, which they are unable to pass through. The ghosts, like the hospital itself, have been abandoned.

NORTH CAROLINA

KISSIE SYKES
CHERRY POINT NAVAL HOSPITAL,
4389 BEAUFORT ROAD,
HAVELOCK

KISSIE SYKES ARRIVED at Cherry Point Naval Hospital late in the summer of 1955. A native of St. Thomas in the United States Virgin Islands, the wife and mother was dead when she got here, but you wouldn't know it by looking at her.

Kissie's body was being prepared for burial when a wind wrought havoc across the islands, snatching away her ghost. After lingering over Puerto Rico, Hurricane Connie dropped her off at the Marine Corps air station, then known as Cunningham Field, on the Neuse River. Dressed in white, the ghost of Kissie Sykes walked to the hospital, chattering about the safety of her children all the way.

It is no great surprise that a hurricane carried Kissie to Havelock. The history of coastal North Carolina is defined by hurricanes and sunken ships. The first hurricane in the written record in America occurred in June 1586 and was referred to as a "terrible storm" that lasted four days. It ravaged the Outer Banks, effectively ending Sir Francis Drake's attempt to support a recently established settlement called the Roanoke Hundred colony. The storm savaged the coast and sank ships. The devastation during what should have been a pleasant June convinced the colonists on Roanoke Island that they'd had enough of the place later to become North Carolina. Instead of dropping off supplies at the first English attempt at a permanent settlement on the North American continent, Drake carried the entire population of colonial America back home to England.

A second group of English colonists, none of whom had experienced the terrible storm of 1586, was dropped off the next year on Roanoke Island. This second colony managed to disappear on its own, becoming known to history as the Lost Colony.

About 370 years later, a hurricane dropped Kissie along the Neuse River. After quickly discovering there was nothing the doctors at Cherry Point could do for her, Kissie left the naval hospital in her St. Thomas burial shroud. She wandered among the facilities at Cunningham Field. A large number of families lived in military housing there. A dedicated mother, she visited more than a few homes, always checking in on the children to see that they were free from harm.

Kissie soon made her way to the airstrip, perhaps intent on catching a ride back to St. Thomas. Marine pilots saw her often enough that Kissie's ghost became a nuisance to aircraft attempting to depart or land. Everyone talked about the ghost in a white dress crisscrossing the airfield day and night. Pilots aborting a landing or takeoff for whatever other reason used Kissie as an excuse.

In an effort to put an end to the distraction, a corpsman from the hospital suggested the ghost be buried. A detail of marines subsequently dug a grave near the airstrip. They asked Kissie to climb into it. She did, and they covered her up. A headstone was purchased and placed over the grave. It reads, "Kissie Sykes, Age 40 Yrs." Actually, her age was someone's best guess.

That was, for a time, the end of Kissie. A ghost transplanted from St. Thomas by a hurricane was planted by shovel and dirt.

It was the end of Kissie until the Marine Corps air station expanded and needed to move the grave to enlarge its airstrips. In the way of the new flight path, Krissie's grave and headstone were relocated to a small cluster of graves in a burial ground not far away.

The relocation disturbed her rest. She felt she might as well keep moving, if she wasn't going to be allowed to rest. Kissie's ghost returned and is still active at Cherry Point today. More devoted than ever to the welfare of children, she frequently appears when a child is being punished or scolded. She doesn't like it. And she particularly doesn't like men who are mean to children, even if it's for the youngsters' own good.

Dare to scold a child at Cherry Point and Kissie in her white dress is instantly there. If you're hollering at the kid, Kissie will slap your face to have you settle down. If the child isn't yours and you're a man, Kissie really gets going with a hard slap and a kick or two.

Late at night when all is still and the children are safe in bed in base housing, Kissie drops by. She silently enters children's bedroom and leaves. Should a child be awake, Kissie talks to him or her in a soft, lilting Caribbean accident. When the child falls back to sleep, Kissie leaves.

Recent developments at the air station suggest Kissie has become overwhelmed by the increase in population at Cherry Point. At last count, more than forty-nine thousand people live and work there, including active-duty and retired marines, their families and children, and a small civilian work force.

A marine corporal stationed at Cherry Point in 2012 reported a troubling encounter he and his wife experienced in base housing. Up late to watch television after his wife had gone to bed, the corporal heard his name shouted from the bedroom. He rushed in to find his shaken wife sitting up in bed with the blankets pulled to her chin. She was staring at a spot in the room. When she calmed down, she told the corporal she had seen a man standing in front of the closet, wearing a World War II uniform.

The serviceman immediately went to bed, in part because he thought his wife was having an "episode" and needed him there. He woke up an hour later to hear a deep male voice saying, "He's not a bad boy." The corporal assumed the ghost was referring to their newly purchased beagle puppy. The puppy, still being housebroken, had been scolded earlier in the day for not making it outside in time. In fact, the corporal had called the puppy a bad boy.

On another occasion, the corporal's wife went to bed with the beagle asleep on the floor beside her. The apparition of a man in an outdated uniform returned. Upon its disappearance, his wife heard a deep male voice say, "We won't always be here to protect you." This occurred the evening of the day the corporal had received transfer orders.

The experience of the young corporal and his wife suggest that Kissie Sykes has recruited other ghosts to help her. This is an exceptionally rare occurrence among known hauntings. Kissie's helpmate seems to have affection for pets and is concerned for their welfare.

Transported by hurricane, refused help in the hospital, and buried where she doesn't want to be, Kissie will likely be unable to find peaceful rest for a long time yet, or at least until parents stop yelling at their kids. Her ghostly recruit, who is known to assist in her vigilance in seeing that children are appropriately and gently cared for, would also have you be kind to animals.

Sometimes, good advice from the afterlife is best delivered as a slap on the face, because some people don't know how to listen.

DANCING DEAD
CHERRY HOSPITAL,
201 STEVENS MILL ROAD,
GOLDSBORO

IT'S TOO EASY TO SAY that something crazy is going on at Cherry Hospital. It is, after all, a facility that treats the mentally ill. But ghosts are making it clear that something from the afterlife has the joint a-jumpin'.

The history of the state hospital in Goldsboro, North Carolina, is a complicated one. The name of the institution changed often over the years. Omitting a few of its official monikers, the hospital has been called the Asylum for Colored Insane, the Eastern North Carolina Insane Asylum for Negroes, the Eastern Asylum for the Colored Race at Goldsboro, and the State Hospital at Goldsboro. In 1961, the inpatient psychiatric facility became Cherry Hospital. That name has stuck—and so have many of its patients buried on the hospital grounds.

Established in 1879 when 171 acres were purchased for an African-American treatment and housing facility, the hospital was enlarged by 1895 with the addition of two three-story patient buildings. In 1929, the facility encompassed 30 buildings on approximately 1,140 acres. By 1976, more than 150 buildings made up the hospital complex.

That's a lot of buildings. And there's a reason. One of the hospital's main purposes was custodial.

Cherry Hospital housed the criminally insane, along with tuberculosis patients and the mentally ill. Early on, being a social or moral outcast was considered sufficient cause for incarceration in a state hospital for the insane. Additional reasons for being committed, according to state records, included both religious laxity and excessive fervor in worship, love affairs, death in the family, jealousy, domestic turmoil, pregnancy, head

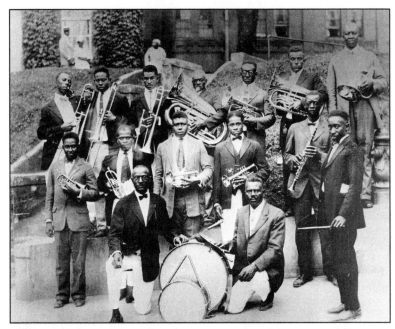

The staff band at Cherry Hospital, formerly known as the "Asylum for Colored Insane" or "the State Hospital" in Goldsboro, North Carolina, photograph circa 1920s
COURTESY OF THE STATE ARCHIVES OF NORTH CAROLINA

injury, sunstroke, fright, destitution, and contagious fever. Others found themselves placed inside a mental hospital for exhibiting the combined symptoms of old age and poverty.

As for treatment, occupational therapy consisted of patients being assigned to assist with fruit, nut, grain, and vegetable growing, livestock production, dairy farming, garment and quilt making, gardening, sawing, and kitchen duties. Sometimes, of course, washing dishes didn't cure clinical depression, at which point recreational therapy took up the slack. Books and magazines, board games, and cards provided opportunities for recreation for the mentally ill at the hospital.

There were also concerts and dances. And it was at these particular therapies that Cherry Hospital excelled. By the early 1900s, it had its own band made up of patients. By the 1920s, the house band was no doubt pumping out jazz for patients on the dance floor. It wasn't long before the musicians taught the cats to swing. Thelonious Monk Sr. came to Cherry Hospital in 1941 and spent the last two decades of his life here. His son, Thelonious Jr., was born in nearby Rocky Mount and often visited his father at the hospital. A 1988 documentary film attributed Thelonious Jr.'s own quirky behavior to mental illness and suggested it may have been inherited from his father. In the film, Thelonious Jr.'s son said that his father sometimes did not recognize him and reported that the pianist and jazz composer was hospitalized on several occasions due to an unspecified mental illness that worsened in the late 1960s.

Tranquilizing medications were widely in use at psychiatric hospitals by 1955. For better or worse, they revolutionized treatment of the mentally ill. This might account for one of the ghostly phenomena at Cherry Hospital—the sound of shuffling feet. At night inside one of the main buildings, faint music from the past can be heard coming from behind closed doors and within locked, unoccupied patient rooms. The music is always accompanied by the rhythmic shuffling of feet across the floor. As the night wears on, the volume of the music increases.

"It gets loud enough you can dance to it in the hall," one of the night nurses at Cherry Hospital said.

At that point, the door to a patient room will be unlocked and swung open. The music and the sound of dancing quickly go away. When the door is closed, a moment of laughter emanates from inside the room, and then all is quiet for the rest of the night.

And in another unoccupied room at Cherry Hospital, the band plays on. And patients from a bygone era get to their feet to dance their lives away.

ZELDA BELLE
HIGHLAND HOSPITAL,
ZILLICOASTREET AND MONTFORD AVENUE,
ASHEVILLE

A GHOST WOMAN walks the streets of the historic Montford neighborhood in Asheville at night, wearing red shoes and carrying a paintbrush. She makes her way through the area of large homes and up Hospital Slope, passing under streetlights as she nears the former site of Highland Hospital.

The apparition appears quite normal from the windows of nearby houses and passing cars. The ghost is clearly recognized as a woman by all who see her, and an attractive woman at that.

"Her hair is quite frizzy," reported a neighborhood resident who approached the ghost while taking her dachshund for a late walk. "Oh, and she smells like smoke."

In a recent interview, the Montford wife said, "The first thing you notice, though, is not the hair. It's the shoes. They're red, bright red."

She also noted that her dachshund didn't bark at the woman. "He usually barks at everyone," she added.

The wife said hello to the frizzy-haired woman as the two approached each other on the nighttime sidewalk.

"She was coming this way, and I was going the other. She stopped when I spoke to her, and so did I. We were almost directly under a streetlight, and I could see her face. She's very pretty. She looked at me as if she might know me and was trying to remember my name. I thought she was going to ask me a question, but instead she just disappeared right where she was standing."

When asked to describe the woman's vanishing act, the resident said,

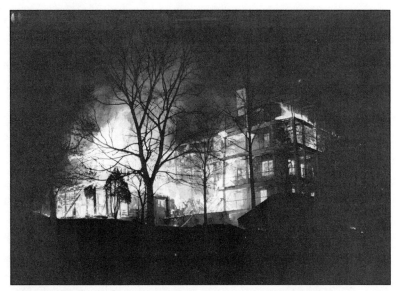

Highland Hospital in flames on March 11, 1948 in Asheville, North Carolina.
Zelda Fitzgerald was one of the victims of the fire.
E. M. BALL PHOTOGRAPHIC COLLECTION, D. H. RAMSEY LIBRARY, SPECIAL
COLLECTIONS, UNIVERSITY OF NORTH CAROLINA AT ASHEVILLE 28804

"It starts at the head and goes down. She just disappears right in front of
you, top to bottom. I remember her red shoes stayed around the longest.
They sort of glowed."

The well-known ghost is referred to as "Zelda Belle" by Asheville residents. If left undisturbed, she stops on the rise near the old hospital site
and paints the air in front of her with her artist's brush. She looks at times
as if she is conducting an unseen, unheard orchestra with her strokes.
Some claim she is painting pictures of flowers and apple trees. An hour
to two later, as morning nears, she walks down the sloping sidewalks and
disappears before dawn.

Zelda Belle is the ghost of one of Asheville's most famous residents.

Born Zelda Sayre in Montgomery, Alabama, the dark-haired beauty
caught a disease at an early age that the doctors in Asheville were unable

to cure. It was called being a Southern belle.

Those who live in Dixie recognize the symptoms of "Southern Belleism"—also known as "the Deadly Sugar"—at a glance. Little girls catch it when they first try on their mamas' fancy dresses and promenade in front of a mirror, wearing a glittering faux glamour and sequined high heels. They catch it in their toes, and it crawls right up their knees, which, according to some, accounts for the invention of the Charleston, a popular dance of the 1920s, named after one of the twinkling cities that are ground zero for Southern Belleism.

Once it takes hold, the affliction cannot be wiped away by slapping at your legs. Zelda described the harrowing advance of Southern Belleism best when she wrote, "I am really only myself when I'm somebody else whom I have endowed with these wonderful qualities from my imagination."

Twenty years before Margaret Mitchell introduced the world to Scarlett O'Hara in *Gone with the Wind*, Zelda Sayre was already demonstrating as severe a case of Southern Belleism as has ever been seen. The disease, as it surges through the body, takes over one's bones and brain. In Zelda's case, famously so.

In the sultry and genteel environment of upper-class Montgomery, Zelda was an icon and a smoldering flame. She wore short skirts, smoked cigarettes, danced "naked" in a lily pond (by wearing a flesh-colored swimsuit), and spent far too much time being courted by boys.

The boys, of course, never really had a chance. But that didn't stop them from trying. A secret society called Zeta Sigma was created at Auburn University in 1919. Its pledges were required to swear an oath of devotion to Zelda. The initiation requirement was traveling to Montgomery to ask Zelda out on a date.

Oddly, the Deadly Sugar does not in its initial stages, which last for years, steal a woman's beauty, as do so many other contagious diseases. In fact, severe cases of Southern Belleism are known to create some of the cutest faces you've ever seen. Zelda was definitely one of those. By all accounts, including her own, she was the preeminent belle of Montgomery. And she wasn't just the belle of the ball. Zelda was the whole dang party.

"All I want to be is very young always and very irresponsible," Zelda wrote, "and . . . be happy and die in my own way to please myself."

She proved quite accomplished at the first part of her wish. But no disease is as much fun as it sounds. Southern Belleism is a dire diagnosis. Zelda died trapped in an addiction to self.

The disease also kills others—those who are charming enough, handsome enough, accomplished enough, and wealthy enough to become the center of attention of a Southern belle. After years of marriage to a carrier of the disease, famous Jazz Age writer F. Scott Fitzgerald, who referred to Zelda as "the first flapper," succumbed to alcoholism a few days before Christmas in 1940.

It is generally safe, and socially acceptable, to be attracted to someone with advanced Southern Belleism. The curse occurs when a Southern belle becomes attracted to you. The proper treatment for those who succumb to the charms of someone with Southern Belleism is laid out in *Gone With the Wind* in the actions taken by Rhett Butler. No matter how entangled one might become with a victim of the Deadly Sugar, the only cure is to leave.

Sadly, Mitchell hadn't yet written her exposé of Southern Belleism when Scott, a Northerner, met Zelda after dropping out of Princeton in 1918 to join the army. He was stationed at Camp Sheridan, just outside Montgomery. They married in 1920. Zelda gave birth to their daughter, Scottie, in 1921.

Zelda was certainly no dummy. She wrote a book or two—after claiming her husband had plagiarized her diaries in order to write his novels. She also drank from life's cup to the fullest, having lived in Paris and on the Riviera, and having fallen in love with a dashing young French pilot while her husband banged away on a book called *The Great Gatsby.* Yet she was still unfulfilled. So she shuttled off her daughter to boarding school and took up ballet.

At twenty-seven, Zelda the belle discovered she was too old to become a star. She took matters into her own hands. While riding in a car driven by her husband, she seized the wheel from Scott and attempted to force the vehicle off a cliff.

It would have been a glamorous, fiery death. But it was not to be.

Her actions did, however, provide a wake-up call for Zelda. She checked herself into a mental hospital. Soon unsatisfied there, she transferred herself to a second hospital, and then a third. "It's dreadful," she wrote of her experience. "It's horrible. What is to become of me?"

Back in the United States, Zelda was admitted to a clinic at Johns Hopkins, where her doctor found no signs of illness, mental or otherwise. The Deadly Sugar, at that time, was not often recognized by doctors in the Northern states.

Zelda returned to the South. In 1936, she came to Highland Hospital in Asheville, where she checked herself in for treatment, which included all sorts of things. Most effective for Zelda was electroshock therapy, and sometimes a treatment called insulin shock, in which coma was induced by repeated, massive injections of insulin. She preferred the former.

She became addicted. Crazy, isn't it? Also known as electroconvulsive therapy, the treatment induces seizures to provide relief from psychiatric illnesses. It's kind of like dancing real fast while lying down. Except it hurts. Although now used as a last line of intervention, electroshock therapy was a standard menu item at Highland. The treatment typically involved multiple administrations, given two or three times per week until a patient, as if by magic, was no longer nervous or depressed.

Zelda repeatedly checked herself into Highland whenever she felt her Southern Belleism had reached the point of emergency. "The trouble with emergencies," she wrote, "is that I always put on my finest underwear and then nothing happens."

Maybe it isn't so difficult to understand an addiction to something that hurts like crazy and puts one's body into convulsions. Remember the first time you ate jalapeños? You recovered and eventually did it again. Electroshock is like going for a roller-coaster ride in your head.

Recovery from the electrically induced convulsions meant staying on at Highland for a few weeks of strolling the neighborhood and painting canvasses. Sometimes, Zelda played tennis. The respite also provided her an escape from the responsibility of having a daughter. And she needn't bother with Scott any longer. He was already dead from the plague of Southern Belleism.

Late at night on March 10, 1948, Zelda found herself, in a hospital gown and something short of her finest underwear, waiting upstairs at Highland for her next electroshock treatment. The therapy was administered at night so the sudden surge in electricity usage wouldn't compete with normal daytime use. Highland, like other mental institutions, had blown more than a few fuses figuring out the proper scheduling.

A fire broke out in the kitchen of the hospital on the hill at the northern end of Montford Avenue. The Asheville fire chief on the night the four-story hospital burned was named, in an odd quirk of circumstance, J. C. Fitzgerald. When he and his seasoned firefighters arrived shortly after one in the morning, they found the building thoroughly in flames. Crews immediately went to work pulling lines, but there was nothing they could do to rescue anyone from the upper story. Patients there were unable to escape, due in part to being heavily medicated but more so because they were locked for the night in rooms with bars on the windows.

Zelda, whose presence at Highland was voluntary, and eight others were dead when the fire was over.

Nervous disorders were a popular diagnosis of the time for those of the gentler sex. Even today, a full 70 percent of electroconvulsive therapy patients are women. But there was one prominent exception among important American writers—Ernest Hemingway, a sometimes close friend of F. Scott Fitzgerald's. At one point, Zelda stated that her husband was actually in love with Hemingway.

Hemingway committed suicide in 1961 shortly after undergoing a series of electroshock treatments at the Mayo Clinic. He is reported by biographer A. E. Hotchner to have complained about the therapy, "Well, what is the sense of ruining my head and erasing my memory, which is my capital, and putting me out of business? It was a brilliant cure but we lost the patient."

Being consumed by fire might be considered a somewhat more glamorous death than putting a shotgun to one's head and pulling the trigger, as did Hemingway. Burning to death is almost ballet in comparison. "Death is the only real elegance," Zelda once wrote.

Throw in a ghost wearing a pair of red shoes on a late-night sidewalk in Montford and what you have is nearly a dance. Zelda Belle has, despite her lifelong bout of Southern Belleism, found a way to grace Asheville with a small and enduring touch of elegance. She is Deadly Sugar consumed in flames.

OTHER NORTH CAROLINA SIGHTINGS

ABERDEEN

The abandoned Pinehurst Convalescent Center, known to most locals as simply "the old nursing home," is hidden in a circle of trees off N.C. 5 just west of Fort Bragg. A victim of vandalism and decay, the sprawling one-story structure was built as a hotel in 1927 and converted to a nursing home in 1951. Of the many aged patients who lived in the identical rooms, at least one remains. He sits in a chair fashioned of PVC pipe with a small wheel at the bottom of each leg. Thieves reportedly have stolen the oddly constructed mobile chair, but it always soon returns. The ghost of the now-deceased patient goes where the chair goes. Those who drop by the closed facility will find the chair in one of the abandoned patient rooms. On their way out of the building, they'll note that the chair has moved seemingly on its own to the other side of the room.

BANNER ELK

Lees-McRae College, a private four-year institution, is noted for its altitude and its buildings constructed of native stones. At 3,720 feet above sea level, it is the highest college or university east of the Mississippi. Lees-McRae was birthed as the first expansion site of the New Opportunity School for Women, a foundation that helps educate and employ women in Appalachia. In its early years, the college accepted chickens, pigs, grain, and other crops in exchange for education costs.

Students housed on the fourth floor of Tate Dormitory share residence with the ghost of Emily, a young girl who died while the building still served as the local hospital. A victim of tuberculosis, Emily succumbed to the disease at age twelve. Her grave at nearby Banner Elk Presbyterian Church is marked with a headstone inscribed, "She is not dead but sleeping."

Apparently, Emily has taken the inscription to heart. She makes her presence known in the dorm through benign antics one would expect of a girl not yet a teenager. She rolls a ball down the fourth-floor hallway and giggles uncontrollably. She is also fond of making the sounds of a rooster's crowing at an early hour. Her farm impressions are, as always, punctuated by fits of giggling.

Famous among dorm residents for at times making it impossible to study or sleep, Emily has of late become an excuse for students who fail to perform up to class standards. One student unable to turn in a research paper on the day it was due told her professor, "The ghost ate my homework."

CHARLOTTE

Founders Hall in downtown Charlotte was built on the site of the city's former medical school. In the mid-1800s, the body of a young girl stolen from a grave in nearby Salisbury was brought to the medical school for study and dissection. A grave disturbed and a body desecrated, let alone dissected, are almost certain to create a lasting ghost.

Evidence of a presence is seen to this day in the city-center building. The handprints of a young person are often discovered in the morning, once housekeepers have completed their shifts. The prints cross the marble floor of the entry to Founders Hall, continue up the wall above the reach of a little girl, and continue still until they touch the ceiling. Clearly, the hands were severed from their arms at some point during dissection.

Sometimes called Lucy, although no one knows the unfortunate girl's name for sure, the ghost appears to be seeking her way out of the building. It is more likely that Lucy is a ghost attempting to escape her past, which is, of course, hands-down impossible.

DURHAM

Watts Hospital was Durham's first. Established in 1895 and relocated in 1909 to an expanded site at the intersection of Club Boulevard and Broad Street, the hospital closed in 1976. After the Spanish Mission–style facilities were remodeled in 1980, the campus became the North Carolina School of Science and Mathematics, a boarding school for academically talented students from across the state.

Someone smart died at the former hospital and has returned to the grounds to assist students. Jokingly named Lloyd, the helpful ghost appears over the shoulders of students who are studying in their residential quarters late at night. The ghost's presence is neither seen nor heard, but rather felt. It has been described by students as an uncomfortable sense that someone is watching and about to touch them. The sense soon overwhelms students to the point of stopping what they're doing and turning around in their chairs to make sure no one is there.

The effect of a visit from Lloyd is simple. When a student returns to the work at hand, whatever difficult problem or concept was the focus of study is immediately solved or understood.

Lloyd may or may not be able to read minds. But the ghost can read notes and books and solve complicated formulas in a flash.

JEFFERSON

Jefferson Hospital, a large stone building on McConnell Street, opened in 1939 and served patients until it closed in 1969. Used for county offices for a number of years, the building is now vacant.

The ghost of someone who died at the hospital didn't mind being inside the building as long as it was populated. Now that everyone is gone and the electrical service has been cut off, the ghost apparently wants to go somewhere else, the sooner the better. The building is maintained and in good repair. Those who enter the old hospital usually do so to provide maintenance. When anyone nears the hospital, the ghost starts shouting. When they come inside, the bell on the old elevator—which hasn't been in service for years—starts to ding.

Some ghosts make noise simply because they are there. The ghost in the old Jefferson Hospital seems to want something more.

MORGANTON

Western Carolina Insane Asylum, now Broughton Hospital, was constructed using convict labor. It opened in Morganton in 1883. A new facility scheduled for completion in 2015 will house the hospital departments and patient divisions under one roof. The original hospital structure, now known as the Avery Building, is listed on the National Register of Historic Places. An imposing six-story brick building with an expanded attic and central domed cupola, it will continue in service.

The building is considered one of the most haunted structures in the state. Ghosts have been active here for more than a hundred years. With one exception, the ghosts are apparitions of former patients who draw themselves from swirls of mist into the appearance of full-bodied individuals. One ghost, however, is quick to get to know new nurses at the hospital. She calls them by name when they are alone. Never seen, this ghost may merely desire that staffers know she is there.

OTEEN

The ghost of a wobbly headed woman walks the grounds near the abandoned nurses' residential building at Charles George VA Medical Center in the community of Oteen, which is now part of Asheville. The large, multistory, empty building is imposing, but not as imposing as the ghost who lives there. Unable to lift her head from one shoulder except to have it flop onto the other, the ghost is said to be that of a nurse who, disappointed in love, hanged herself from a window of the structure.

RALEIGH

Originally the North Carolina Insane Asylum, Dorothea Dix Hospital in Raleigh admitted its first patient in 1856. Soon after that, a cemetery was set aside on the property. The first internment there was in 1859. The three-acre "Dix Hill" cemetery, which contains at least nine hundred graves, provided ground for its last customer in the 1970s.

The only graves with tombstones were those of the few patients at the asylum whose families possessed the means. Due to erosion and neglect, the cemetery became filled with unmarked graves and depressions in the ground known as "coffin hollows." In later years, trucks hauling garbage were driven over the cemetery's edges on their way to and from a nearby landfill. In the 1970s, hospital employees used kitchen forks to prod for the location of caskets that had drifted during a heavy rain.

Natural deterioration is anticipated following death. A little erosion here and there is something a body might anticipate after burial. But the trucks loaded with fetid garbage were another thing altogether, an insult and injury that disturbed the dead.

Ghosts walk the graveyard at night. Small lights have appeared in pairs since the 1970s. And though steps have been taken to clean up the cemetery and make things right, the lights are still seen. They mark the boundaries of where it is unwise to trespass if you intend to respect the dead. As with all cemeteries, you should enter—or inter, whichever comes first—with appropriate care.

ROXBORO

An unlikely ghost inhabits a restaurant in Roxboro.

A hospital train that saw service during the War Between the States was retired alongside a train car used to transport bodies. They sat for several years, empty of all but ghosts. They were later moved to the station at Roxboro and are now used as dining rooms at a restaurant there.

Diners who enjoy ghostly visits should choose seating inside the body car. A mirror on the wall reflects the image of a Confederate officer who has become known as a "thirty-second ghost." To see him, diners need to stand directly in front of the mirror. But they shouldn't tarry. The ghost is looking at himself and will disappear instantly should his view be blocked for too long.

STATESVILLE

The old Carpenter-Davis Hospital on South Center Street has long been closed. Built in 1920, the three-story brick building is haunted by the ghosts of former patients who died there. A favorite hunting ground for paranormal investigators, many of whom are themselves not quite normal, the building is haunted by roving cold spots created by the dead. Everyone who enters feels cold even in summer. Additionally, voices of the dead murmur over empty cribs stored in the basement. Whether you hear ghost voices or not, you'll hear your teeth chatter if you stay in one place very long.

While some ghosts manifest their presence by creating masses of frigid air that are experienced when people walk through specific areas, the cold spots inside the old Carpenter-Davis Hospital come to find visitors. Some ghosts, it turns out, are people hunters. They slip into living bodies as one might slip into a warm coat or a cozy bed.

SOUTH CAROLINA

GHOST DELIVERY
SPARTANBURG REGIONAL MEDICAL CENTER, 110 EAST WOOD STREET, SPARTANBURG

MELISSA WAS COMPLETELY fouling up her first semester at Wofford College. Something was wrong with the whole world. Her grandmother died the day after classes started. She was buried following a closed-casket viewing and service. Melissa missed critical classes. She missed the very beginning, the most important initial steps of her possibly being an A student in college. Not so long ago, acing her college classes had been Melissa's dream.

Melissa and her grandmother were close. At least they had been. It was impossible to say goodbye to a closed box, the freshman learned. It was doubly awful for another reason. Melissa's grandmother had lived her last two weeks in the hospital, during which time she was sent home to die and then rushed back to the hospital in an ambulance. All the while, she refused to see her granddaughter.

Two weeks earlier, Melissa's mother had laid down the law. Visiting her grandmother was forbidden.

"She doesn't want you to see her like that, Melissa, and you won't. It's her dying wish. Don't you understand?"

"No," Melissa said. She was crying. "I don't care how bad she looks. I don't care!"

"She wants you to remember her like she was before this final stage." Her mother handed her a tissue.

"I don't want to remember her, Momma. I want to talk to her. And tell her I love her and always will. I want to thank her."

"You can write a card, dear. They'll read it to her."

Melissa shook her head. She sobbed. Her mother didn't understand.

"This is hard on everyone, Melissa. Don't make it any harder. She wouldn't want that."

The hospital staff wouldn't let her grandmother wear her teeth. The frail old woman was being fed through a tube surgically placed into her stomach. She was covered with lesions. She drooled. And they wouldn't let her wear her wig.

Melissa didn't care. But her grandmother did.

On her way to her brand-new life as a college coed living in Greene Residence Hall, a Wofford dormitory on Church Street, Melissa decided to break the rules. Her family was wrong. Her grandmother was wrong. Her grandmother was weak and out of her mind on drugs. She didn't know what she wanted and what she didn't want.

And Melissa was tired of crying. With a U-Haul trailer attached to the back of her car, she drove to her grandmother's house. It was locked. A neighbor said the elderly woman had been taken back to the hospital.

Spartanburg Regional was next door to Wofford. Once there, Melissa was told by three different people that her grandmother wanted no visitors.

She carried her things into the dorm. She met her roommate, who was nice enough but seemed scared of Melissa, for some reason. Melissa installed a bracketed shelf on the wall.

By the time her grandmother's death was weeks old, Melissa was barely making it to classes. She couldn't study. She couldn't concentrate. Melissa wanted to leave. Not just school, she wanted to leave it all, to go somewhere and sit alone for a long time.

Melissa tied her hair in a ponytail, quit wearing makeup, and wept until her face was heavily blotched. Once when she started to brush her teeth, Melissa glanced in the mirror and stopped. She looked horrible. She stepped into the shower with her clothes on, but the warm water only made her cry harder.

Melissa's roommate made a habit of not staying in the dorm room.

She'd sneak in late when the grieving freshman was already in bed, pretending to be asleep. Sometimes, Melissa saw her in the morning, but not for long. She barely remembered the girl's name.

One evening, alone, disturbed, and unable to think, Melissa heard a siren. She often heard ambulances on their way to Spartanburg Regional. Their whoops and screams were part of the background noise at Wofford. But this one was different. It was right outside her dorm in the middle of the night.

Soon, she heard a knock on the door. Melissa peeped through the hole. A man she had never seen before was standing there, dressed in white.

"Yes?" she asked, opening the door just far enough to talk.

"I have something to tell you," he said. "May I come inside?"

Of course not, she thought. A man she had never seen before knocking on her door at night? Melissa said later that she would never have opened the door to a stranger, not under any circumstances. But the man had a purpose other than to accost her. She could sense it in some strange way and felt safe. Melissa opened the door. Her hand was steady and not shaking.

He walked in like he was there to fix something. The man wore white pants, white shoes, and a short-sleeved white shirt with a bowtie. He looked like someone from the 1950s selling ice cream at the drugstore.

"I'm with the ambulance out front," he said.

"From the hospital?" Melissa asked, closing the door behind him. "Did my roommate call for help?"

"I'm not here to take anyone to the hospital."

He smiled and sat on the roommate's bed, his knees facing Melissa's. She sat down across from him. He smiled again, and Melissa began to cry. She understood without asking for more information.

"Is my grandmother with you?"

"She will be," he told her. "She's right outside, but I have a message for you first. From your grandmother."

Melissa lifted her head to listen. Her face was streaked with tears. She tried her best to breathe without sobbing.

"She wants you to know that she is fine. She is happy and safe. Your grandmother wants you to stop crying. She said there is nothing for you to cry about. And there's one last thing."

Melissa shuddered and choked on her tears. She couldn't help it. Her body trembled and quaked. She shook like a tiny leaf caught in an electric fan.

"Her finally message is that she wants you to go back to class and do well in school. It's time. Your grandmother said that your time is now."

There was a loud bang in the room. The sound was so solid that Melissa was certain her shelf had fallen and the unabridged dictionary her grandmother had bought her for college had landed on the floor. She looked. The shelf and her books were still there.

"It starts now, Melissa," the man said.

Melissa stopped crying as the room filled with the smell of White Shoulders, her grandmother's favorite perfume.

Melissa felt a weight on the bed behind her. She could not turn around to look. Her grandmother didn't want her to. Then she felt a comforting hand on her shoulder.

The man who had driven the ambulance to bring her grandmother's ghost to Melissa's dorm stood. He cleared his throat. The weight lifted from the bed. The hand was gone. And so was the messenger ghost. Melissa listened to the siren as the ambulance drove away. She was left with the faint scent of her grandmother's perfume.

Her body felt like a washcloth you twist in your hands until all the water is gone, and twist one more time to be sure. She slept soundly for the first night since coming to Wofford. Off and on, sirens yelled their approach to the medical center next door. Melissa dreamed it was her grandmother singing as she worked on a recipe in the kitchen with Melissa standing next to her, a young girl wrapped in an apron that was too big.

Melissa made almost all A's that semester. And the next. And the ones that followed. She and her roommate became best friends. She never cried for her grandmother again. It didn't matter that Melissa hadn't seen her when she wanted to. She'd seen her grandmother at her best.

And her grandmother was there to see her graduate. The smell of her perfume said so.

ALICIA FLEW
I-26 REST AREA, NEWBERRY

On a warm night in July, the usual fog drifted across the interstate that slides through the outer edges of Sumter National Forest. Alicia May Goodwin, who'd been seeking a ride, was found stranded and badly injured in the median of I-26 near the Newberry rest area. A couple stopped to help her. Alicia told them she'd been hit by a car.

Ambulances and a fire rescue unit were soon on the scene. The twenty-seven-year-old woman required immediate emergency transport.

A crew of three—a flight nurse, a flight paramedic, and a pilot—arrived from Spartanburg Regional Medical Center. The medevac team circled overhead, then descended. The craft's "night sun" searchlight was on to improve visibility in the fog, which was thickest above the trees. It landed in front of a fire truck in the eastbound lanes of I-26. The hit-and-run victim was stable as she was carried to the miniature emergency hospital, which readied for liftoff after spending less than ten minutes on the ground.

The chopper lifted over the highway and crossed the westbound lanes of I-26. It gained altitude to climb above the trees and turned toward Spartanburg.

It didn't get farther than that. The helicopter pitched forward, fell into the trees, and crashed with a violent explosion. Witnesses reported hearing a boom and seeing a flash of light from the heavily wooded area where the Bell 407 helicopter went down.

All aboard were dead.

Although Alicia flew, she now walks. Travelers on I-26 sometimes mistake the momentary burst of light in the trees at five-thirty in the morning for lightning.

Just as often on foggy mornings, they mistake Alicia's ghost for a living person. Alicia asks for a lift when a vehicle stops on the shoulder of I-26. Those who have met the ghost hiking through the fog on the interstate say she looks as normal as anyone else. Another, smaller flash of light comes as she tries to open the door when offered a ride. When the light goes out, Alicia is gone.

Angry perhaps that she cannot leave the scene of her death, Alicia isn't just another hitchhiker asking for a lift. She is asking for a life.

Although drivers along I-26 near Newberry have the opportunity every morning at five-thirty, the best advice is not to offer the ghost a ride. Truckers pausing at the rest stop to catch a few winks before first light often trade stories. The most popular says that if Alicia ever manages to get the door of your vehicle open, you will die in a brilliant flash of light.

Ask around, if you dare, the next time you're traveling through South Carolina on I-26 in the vicinity of mile marker 64. Just be careful who you talk to. If it's the ghost of Alicia Goodwin, your questions could cost you your life. Like the fog, she is always drifting. But she never gets far. Thus far, anyway.

THE LENGTHENING TREE
BROWNS FERRY ROAD, GEORGETOWN

DR. LYDIA CURED HER PATIENTS by inches. The doctor's renown extended far beyond what is today Georgetown, South Carolina, and indeed the entire continent.

She specialized in an area of medicine scoffed at by the more educated doctors of Europe and the newly founded United States. But that didn't keep her from being sought out by those in need of her services. Quite the contrary. Many came from abroad, crossing the Atlantic at their own peril. It was an expense they had best be able to afford, since the doctor accepted payment only in gold.

Late of Liverpool, England, Myron Addison decided he would be "Lord Myron" upon reaching the Bay of Winyah in South Carolina. Let the curious wonder how a man his size might merit that title.

Lord Myron was sick of the curious and their stares, weary of the taunts of children. Mostly, he was tired of being short.

He was about to become a man of height. A woman of Prince George Parish, Winyah, was going to see to it for him. Her brochure guaranteed it.

Lord Myron, a short man in a checkered vest and dark blue britches, hired a wagon at Brown's Ferry. The driver loaded Lord Myron's two satchels in the back. Rather than facing the indignity of asking for the assistance he would require to ride in the wagon seat, the Lord of Liverpool climbed into the back and sat between his bags.

"Dr. Lydia's," he told the driver.

The man rubbed his stubbled chin. "Do you mean the parish witch?"

After sleeping in the attic of the doctor's small house at the edge of the indigo fields south of the parish, Lord Myron allowed Dr. Lydia to place a poultice on his forehead.

"The herbs inform the brain that it is time to tell the body to grow," she explained.

Shortly, she ushered him outdoors to undergo the extension of his abbreviated body.

Lord Myron discovered Dr. Lydia's hospital was her backyard. The treatment table was a ladder under an oak tree. And a rope of wound jute. He half-expected leather straps and chains and a large wooden wheel.

Following a series of trial-and-error adjustments and some assistance from Lord Myron, the doctor managed to position the ladder rungs at the perfect height. She tied one of the patient's wrists to a notched branch of the tree. His feet remained on the ladder rung she specified.

One arm lifted over his head and seemingly held tightly in place by its binding, Lord Myron was told to reach his foot to the rung below and to holler for the doctor when he accomplished the impossible feat.

"Tell the body to extend," Dr. Lydia instructed. "With the mind," she added, pointing to her head.

The patient unbuttoned his vest with one hand and waited for his mind to achieve the miracle. It had happened for others, and it would happen for him. Lowly Mr. Addison would become Lord Myron.

He watched the birds for a spell, then lowered one toe. It wouldn't reach. He studied the progress of the slaves working in the indigo fields. He groaned now and then. His arm was sore. When he reached his toe a second time, it touched the lower step. But he couldn't quite stand on it yet. Still, he was already taller.

The cure was not a miracle by any stretch. The jute had been wound into rope loosely, allowing it to give over time. And it was tied in a clever way so that his wrist moved lower in the loops of the knot that surrounded it. The branch was wrapped thrice in the rope. The inner loop tightened around the oak by the pull of the Englishman's weight. This allowed the outer loop to slacken and droop but still hold his wrist as tightly as it had when first knotted. Besides, he needed to move only an inch and a half to reach the next step.

The jute slowly gave way to gravity, time, and the pull of his body. And it wasn't long before Lord Myron was a little bit taller. He shouted with joy as his entire foot reached the rung below. The Englishman was so excited that he nearly kicked the ladder out from under him.

"Your trouser leg is shorter on this side," the doctor said. "Tomorrow, we do the other side. And then we start over, and you will grow more. You can be as tall as you desire."

Or as tall as he had gold coins. She accepted the first payment and climbed the ladder to untie him.

Yes, his arm was sore, but it was longer. And so was one leg. He noticed it when he walked.

Dr. Lydia made tea that afternoon and served it with thick chunks of bread dipped in milk. For supper, they ate squirrel stew with potatoes.

Before he climbed his way to bed, she offered him a pipe of tobacco.

"Tomorrow is one more coin," she told him.

Lord Myron agreed.

The next day, they did it again, this time with the other arm tied to the branch of the oak.

Lord Myron, pleased with his two shorter trouser legs, happily paid his gold sovereign to Dr. Lydia. It was a mere token to him. He would stay for weeks of treatments. He would be six feet tall, he decided, before he left America. Or five-foot-ten at a minimum. Either way, he'd need new clothes. And a walking stick long enough to reach the ground when he held it.

That night, men from the church came with violent complaints against Dr. Lydia. They shouted that she was a witch. Lord Myron struggled against the intruders but soon collapsed, bruised and short of breath. The mob of determined parishioners carried her to the tree, where they proved to be short of mercy.

Dr. Lydia was hanged from the oak branch. She stood on the ladder, strangling. Members of the mob used torches to set fire to the ladder. The heat scalded leaves all the way to the top of the oak.

In the name of all things holy, they dropped to their knees and prayed. One rose to his feet to grab the frantic man flailing at their backs.

"No!" Lord Myron screamed as he was thrown to the ground. He kicked with both feet at the soil and sodden leaves. But there was nothing he could do to save the doctor from her fiery fate. He stared in anguished horror at Dr. Lydia, who dangled dead from the treatment tree, her clothes blazing, her skin shriveling from the heat. "No, no, no!"

"Be still in the presence of righteousness, my little man," he was commanded by the group's leader. "Be still or be put still."

Soon, her hair sizzled and the fire went out. Lord Myron wailed. He paused, thinking to wail further.

But then he thought of the gold coins he'd given the doctor. Those, and likely many more, were in the little house somewhere.

Men in town spoke of the small man who had loved her, who had been unable to detect her compact with Satan. When they traveled to the house two days later to preach to him, they found the Englishman gone entirely.

"So much was he in love with her, he killed himself," one speculated.

The others agreed, having witnessed the man throw himself on the ground, having heard his sadness and grief during her brief trial on the tree.

"He threw his body in the bay," another suggested. "There is no other explanation. Indeed, it is a deep sorrow."

"I wonder, brother, what sort of splash he made."

The pious brethren thought better than to laugh at their joke.

They buried her face-down under the tree. In case she should seek to return, as witches sometimes did, Dr. Lydia would be going the wrong way and reach an altogether different destination. It was something short of a Christian burial.

Not far along an old dirt road off S.C. 51 just north of Georgetown, people claim you can still locate Dr. Lydia's hospital tree. It's most easily found in the evening as shadows lengthen. The gnarled oak stands taller than the trees surrounding it. To reach the aged tree, you need only walk a short way.

Dr. Lydia's ghost moans at the time of night of her demise. Hundreds have heard it over the years and report that it is a regular occurrence at the location of her death. Fewer have discovered the grave under the tree, one small portion of which was long ago burned by fire. If you stand on the grave, whether on purpose or by accident, the ghost of the midget-stretcher will holler from under the ground at your feet. It sounds like an echo. Her spirit will hold you in place. No matter how you stretch and lean, you cannot leave until you scream. A scream breaks the spell.

As for Lord Myron, no record exists of his return passage to Liverpool. Some say he grew a long mustache and invested heavily in indigo. Having fallen short of his original goal, he increased his stature by increasing his wealth.

OTHER SOUTH CAROLINA SIGHTINGS

AIKEN

Annie's Inn, formerly a doctor's residence and county clinic in the Montmorenci district, is a large Greek Revival two-story home built in the 1830s as the primary house on a two-thousand-acre plantation. The original third story was destroyed by cannon fire during the War Between the States. In the late 1800s and through the turn of the twentieth century, the house served as a hospital. A young girl thought to be the doctor's daughter died there. Prior to her death, however, she seems to have been given the run of the central stairway. Her voice is still heard today—downstairs if you're at the top, upstairs when you're at the bottom.

"It's just the eeriest thing," says current owner Scottie Ruark, who's operated the house as an inn since 1984. "It's an actual voice, and it's scary."

Recent reports of the aural haunting at Annie's Inn indicate the girl's voice is most often heard calling out for her mother. One wonders how long it was before Mom stopped running up and down the stairs every time the little girl called for her.

BEAUFORT

Beaufort Memorial Hospital, on Port Royal Island, is haunted by a pair of ghosts, one of whom brings comfort to patients in the form of prayer. The comfort comes after the patients recover from seeing a Confederate soldier standing at the foot of the bed. That apparition is accompanied by a woman, who is left behind as the soldier vanishes. She stands next to the bed and recites a prayer.

"I saw her standing there praying," a former patient said. "And I felt complete peace."

There truly is someone other than hospital personnel watching over patients at Beaufort Memorial.

CHARLESTON

The old Marine Hospital on Franklin Street, a National Historic Landmark, was completed in 1833 as a city facility to treat sick and injured sailors and provide them with quarters while they recovered—or failed to do so. Consisting of two stories above a raised basement, the subtly Gothic structure is haunted by a ghost, apparently trapped in the basement, who sings sea shanties at odd hours in a drunken, raspy voice. The old salt apparently broke into a supply of liquor in the basement and drank himself to death.

A favorite song in the ghost's repertoire is "Anne Boleyn with Her Head Tucked In."

CHARLESTON

A nurse prone to accidents haunts the grounds of the Charleston Naval Hospital Historic District.

Sarah Louise Chapman joined the service soon after the bombing of Pearl Harbor. Stationed at the hospital, she quickly earned a reputation for falling over her own feet. Sarah Lou, in fact, could manage to fall when standing still. Once, while preparing to administer a shot in a treatment room, she turned to face her patient. Uttering the single word "Oops," and without taking a single step, the nurse folded into a pile of legs on the floor. In an attempt to break her fall, Sarah Lou injected herself.

Her accomplishment was mentioned in the base newspaper the following week, as were other incidents in subsequent weeks. Thereafter, anyone who goofed up at the Charleston Naval Base was said to have "pulled a Sarah Lou."

The hapless—and generally harmless—nurse left the service at the end of World War II. She married and had children. Now deceased, Sarah Lou has returned to the location of her service. Her ghost appears regularly in the historic district, dressed in a World War II nurse's uniform. She is most often seen tumbling down the steps while heading in or out of buildings. Occasionally, she appears on the sidewalk, stumbling forward with her navy-issue purse swung far out from her body for balance. The

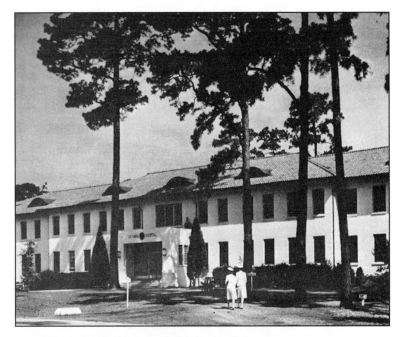

Naval Hospital in Charleston, South Carolina, in 1948
OFFICIAL U.S. NAVY PHOTOGRAPH

apparition vanishes once her stumble or tumble is complete, but never without witnesses hearing a female voice say, "Oops."

COLUMBIA

The University of South Carolina campus is haunted by two visually startling ghosts, especially near the tunnel entrances to the catacombs used as hospitals by both Union and Confederate forces during the War Between the States.

In the area of Rutledge Chapel, the apparition of a soldier who suffered a musket shot to the forehead exits the tunnels. He has become known as "the Three-Eyed Ghost" among students and faculty, who have mistaken his wound for an eye.

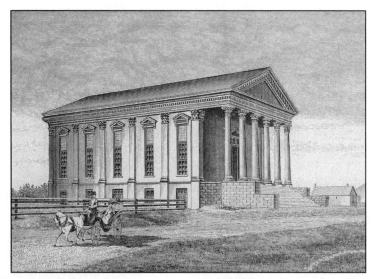

Engraving of Longstreet Theatre in Columbia, South Carolina, circa 1860
COURTESY OF SOUTH CAROLINIANA LIBRARY, UNIVERSITY OF SOUTH CAROLINA,
COLUMBIA, S.C.

Another striking ghost appears outside the Longstreet Theatre. Re-markably, the ghost is a shimmering, mirror-like apparition. Known as "the Silver Ghost," the figure is easily seen at night, reflecting light from an unknown source. Thought to be the ghost of a soldier who suffered severe injuries when a supply of gunpowder ignited, the tall figure rises from the catacombs to escort female students walking alone at night. Al-though the poor fellow's death was likely painful, his afterlife has proven to be long and lustrous.

COLUMBIA

In 1913, a tuberculosis recuperation site was established at Ridge-wood Camp. Patients with TB initially occupied tents and were isolated from the general population. In 1920, the sale of Christmas Seals gener-ated additional funds for the camp, allowing the erection of a few cottage-style structures for quartering patients and public-health nurses. Eventually, a main building was constructed, as were separate facilities for African-American patients. Ridgewood even had its own dairy barn. What it didn't have was a church.

When people in the South can't make it to church, church comes to them. And so does the choir. The former Ridgewood site is haunted by a rather pleasant and altogether enthusiastic hymn singer. Thought to be the spirit of a former visiting choir member, the ghost is more often heard than seen. Accompanied only by the rhythmic clapping of unseen hands, the bluesy female voice makes it all the way through the verses of a traditional church hymn before fading into the Sunday breeze among the trees. The ghost is happy and she knows it.

GEORGETOWN

For unexplained reasons, some ghosts who don't mind being seen prefer not to gaze upon the living. Either that or they don't realize people are present. Such is the case with a ghost at Georgetown Memorial Hospital.

While working for Midway Fire Rescue, an emergency medical technician made numerous trips to Georgetown Memorial, usually late at night or early in the morning. He reported seeing a ghost on three occasions between 2005 and 2007.

"He is slender and appears to be between the ages of eighteen and twenty-two," the EMT said. "His eyes are empty. He has two white orbs where his irises should be."

The rescue worker also noted that the ghost was present when the emergency room was extremely busy.

"On one occasion, I attempted to speak to him, but he never acknowledged me," he said.

Speculation is that the ghost is trapped where he died and doesn't want to be there. He doesn't even want to look at the place.

GREENVILLE

When it rains in Greenville, South Carolina, ghosts leak out of the ground.

All that is left of the former Hopewell Tuberculosis Sanatorium is a few puddles that turn red with blood after a rain. The puddles are located near a memorial bench in Herdklotz Park. Locals suggest the blood is from patients who died at the TB hospital, and that the park bench stands on the site of the institution's former morgue.

ROCK HILL

Rock Hill, a city of sixty-eight thousand, is noted for its four distinctive statues of women, called the *Civitas*, at Gateway Park—and for a bloody ghost who sits outside the emergency room at Piedmont Medical Center.

The hospital is a proud sponsor of the annual South Carolina Strawberry Festival in nearby Fort Mill. Festivities include a pageant that selects as many as three Strawberry Queens each year.

The ghost waiting patiently in a chair outside the emergency room wears a white gown, a tiara, and glossy lipstick. Although she appears ready to smile, she will not respond to questions. Her posture is excellent.

The apparition is that of a Strawberry Festival runner-up who died in the hospital when she mistakenly thought she had suffered no major injury in a car wreck. Unaware she had an artery pierced by a sliver of glass, she became drenched in her own blood when the sliver moved while she adjusted herself in an uncomfortable chair in the waiting area. All the while, she was waiting for her boyfriend to be treated by emergency services.

The young lady maintained her composure while dying. Her ghost sits perfectly upright but vanishes when spoken to.

Were she to respond to the standard pageant question, it is an even bet she would say, "World peace."

TENNESSEE

THE BOX
GREENBRIER RESTAURANT,
370 NEWMAN ROAD,
GATLINBURG

FINDING A HOSPITAL GHOST can be as easy as letting the ghost find you. This particular ghost lives in a lidded box—perhaps the smallest and most common hospital in the country. Such an emergency hospital may already be in your home, the garage workshop, the trunk of your car, the back of your boat, or stored with the camping equipment in your basement or attic.

The ghost is Debbie. The important part of her life story is that she died young. This was way back in time, before cell phones and the Internet, when boys with the means had cassette players in their cars and girls still wore dresses to school. Back when Gerry Rafferty was hanging out on Baker Street and the Bee Gees had Saturday Night Fever, Debbie, unlucky in love, took her own life. She was barely sixteen.

As we age, we learn that, in love, as in most other things, we roll the dice. When we lose, we gather our courage and eventually roll the dice again, hoping that this time chance will turn in our favor. The first roll of the dice of love should never be the last. But kids don't know it. They believe they have only one shot at the thing—one honeysuckle summer, and no more than that.

So when Steve kissed Debbie and Debbie kissed him back, the dice began their tumble. For Debbie, it was eternal love and complete devotion to the boy of her dreams, the future father of her children. He had blond hair and his own car. He had blue eyes, and so did Debbie. He played baseball for the high-school team. He drove Debbie to her summer job at the Greenbrier Restaurant and was in the parking lot, waiting, when her shift was over.

They spent her tips on gas and drove through the warm, starlit nights. They circled through the mountains on ridge roads; they went up and down the main drag in town; they parked. They held hands everywhere they went. And all the while, they talked about what was next for both of them.

Steve said he might have to play in the minors for a season, maybe two.

"I don't care where it is," Debbie told him. "As long as it's with you, I'm there."

The dice, however, were still tumbling. In the South, when the dice of love come up a winner, it's called "throwing roses." Dice are white bones with black eyes. And when they come to a stop at the end of a throw, they never lie. Debbie's dice came up thorns.

Steve stopped showing up. There was no warning, no hint that anything was different. He just wasn't there. In Debbie's heart, she'd lost everything. She didn't even have a heart, she thought. All she had was an empty hole. She was dead inside.

Thorns draw blood. So did Debbie. Her own.

She cut her wrists outside the Greenbrier. She whimpered and cried. Then she cut them again, twisting the knife she'd taken from the kitchen, gouging. Tired of waiting for her blood to pour out, Debbie plunged the blade into her chest. That little trick turned everything red.

In the middle of a summer night, Debbie was sitting with her back against the outside restaurant wall. A coworker who'd stayed late to clean the grease traps saw her in the headlights when he started his car to leave. He left the headlights on and rushed to her side.

When he saw the blood, when she didn't answer him, he unlocked the restaurant and hurried inside. He called the police on the dial phone at the cashier's station. Then he found the box. It was in the kitchen. He ran back to Debbie with the first-aid kit. Kneeling beside her, he flipped the latch and popped the lid open. He heard her moan. It was the last thing Debbie ever said.

The coworker had seen something in a movie and thought he should leave the knife where it was. He tore open adhesive bandages and applied them to Debbie's wrists. Her arms were limp. He wrapped the bandages with white tape he had to tear with his teeth. Her heart wasn't beating. He scrambled through the items in the box. He found tweezers and wondered why. The tube of antibiotic ointment was no good to anyone in an actual emergency.

Little Debbie wasn't breathing. Her eyes were closed. Black mascara streaked her cheeks. The rest of her was covered with blood.

"I can pick her up," he told the uniformed officer when the police arrived. "She doesn't weigh a hundred pounds."

The officer had brought along his own lidded metal box. It was bigger than the one from the restaurant. He opened and closed it without taking anything out.

"Doesn't matter," the officer said. "We may as well wait for the ambulance. One's on its way. We'll let them take the knife out and tell us she's dead. Do you know where her daddy lives?"

When Debbie's body was laid to rest, she didn't go with it. She had a cozier place in which to dwell. Neat, clean, and metal, it was better by far than a wooden crate surrounded by soil and worms.

A first-aid kit is a hospital in a box. The one from the restaurant, some of its contents removed, was offered for a dollar at a yard sale. Every time someone opened it, Debbie moaned. It was set back on the folding table time and time again. But eventually, somebody not paying attention took it home.

The buyer woke that night thinking he heard his wife moaning in her sleep. He touched her gently and said to wake up, that it was only a dream. His wife mumbled, rolled over, and breathed normally. Meanwhile, Debbie watched from the foot of their bed. When the man finally saw her, the first thing he noticed was a knife in her chest. He kicked the covers and yelled for Debbie to go away.

She left but came back the next night while the couple slept. She stood at the foot of their bed and stared, wondering what they had that made love last forever. It wasn't the husband's looks, that was for sure.

He was bald, old, and too fat to play baseball. He burped in his sleep. The couple never held hands.

She stood by their bed night after night to think it over before slipping back into the lidded box. There was plenty for blue-eyed Debbie to learn about love. She had all the time in the world.

The man figured out that the ghost had started showing up when he brought home the used first-aid kit from the yard sale. He asked his wife to get rid of it. She took it to the Holiday Inn in Gatlinburg, where she worked as a reservation clerk. Debbie peeked out of her box from behind the counter when people checked in. She'd roll the dice and choose guests to look in on late at night, when everyone was in bed. She learned a lot that year.

Debbie's ghost is still learning. She's puzzled by one thing.

The first-aid kit is no longer at the Holiday Inn. Too useful to throw away, it circulates among houses and garages and car trunks in Gatlinburg. Someone always takes Debbie home with them. Someone always will. With a little luck, Debbie will figure out love one day and leave the box she's in. Perhaps then she'll find a quiet place in the beyond and rest up for a thousand years from her nights of seeking. Or maybe the dice of life will come up snake eyes for Steve, and Debbie will receive an answer to the question she wants to ask, from the only person who can answer it.

What in the world did I do to make you leave me?

BOILED BONES
NEAR WATER AND RAILROAD STREETS, CHARLESTON

HEAVY RAINS IN THE SPRING of 1867 and the resulting flood of the Hiwassee River washed away the railroad bed outside Charleston, Tennessee. This resulted in the wreck of a steam passenger train of the Cincinnati, Cumberland Gap and Charleston Railroad. The train left the rails and plunged into a steep and flooded ravine. The town was in a state of emergency. Volunteers under the direction of the town doctor recovered numerous bodies from the wreckage, many of whom had drowned.

The remains of a young man wearing a monk's robe and cowl were carried to the doctor's office. Of the bodies, this was the only one left unidentified. The railway had no record of his having been a passenger on the train. A kindly ticket agent may have let him ride without purchasing a fare.

He became an unknown corpse in need of burial. With no known family to pay the cost of internment and no address the town could use to ship the body home, the doctor came up with a viable alternative. He would use the body as a skeleton.

Within a few weeks, the rack of boiled bones occupied a corner of the examination room in the physician's office in town. The doctor referred to it often, pointing out the exact spot on the skeleton where a patient had suffered an injury. He called the skeleton "the Monk."

The doctor died. His practice closed.

The ghost of the monk lingered inside the physician's office, apparently attached in the afterlife to something located there. A variety of tenants occupied the building, but none stayed long. They left once it became clear the place was haunted. More disturbingly, the ghost appeared to be entirely naked.

"And he looks a little wet," one tenant reported.

Though a peaceful ghost, the naked monk was unsettling. The last owner of the building had it demolished in 1932. As the walls came down, two things of interest were discovered. Hidden inside a small sealed-off closet that was once used as a pantry were the monk's brown robe and a rosary that dated to 1867. From the rosary of ebony beads hung a crucifix made of silver.

These were given to the pastor of the local church, along with the skeleton, which had been tucked away in an upper room of the Masonic lodge. The skeleton was subsequently dressed in the monk's robe and buried in the churchyard. Appropriate respects were paid the remains. Pious words were spoken. However, the pastor was not Catholic. He did his best, but the burial was likely not one the young monk would have preferred.

At least his ghost had a place to go other than the site of the torn-down building. And maybe, the pastor hoped, that place was close to heaven.

The ghost was not content with the outcome. He wants to go where he was headed when the train took its plunge outside Charleston. Since 1932, locals have seen him wandering the railroad tracks at the edge of town, seeking passage to another place and time.

The hooded monk walks up and down the tracks, unable to flag a ride. Trains pass right through him. He walks a ways on the tracks. And walks back, waiting all the while to catch a ride on a train that never stops for ghosts.

THICK AS COFFEE
NETHERLAND INN ROAD, KINGSPORT

EVERYONE KNOWS that people die in hospitals. But sometimes leaving a hospital is more dangerous that being there, especially if a foggy road is involved.

Hugh was reading the back pages of the Sears & Roebuck catalog when neighbor Lester Saunders hollered on the front porch that he was coming in the door.

"Don't shoot!" Lester yelled. "Charlie's driven the Lizzie off the road. They took him to the hospital. We better get you there."

Unsure what to take with him, Hugh grabbed the enameled coffeepot off the stove and followed Lester out the door. Hugh set the pot on the floorboard between his feet while Lester started the Chevy FB-40 sedan. They powered along Netherland Inn Road on the Chevy's steel wheels, which Lester insisted could drive everywhere wooden-spoke wheels couldn't.

"Headlights could be brighter," Hugh said. The fog was murder along the Holston River this time of night. It was thick as coffee. "Is he dead?"

"Haven't heard a thing except he's at the hospital," Lester replied.

When they reached the hospital, Hugh climbed out of the idling Chevy, coffeepot in hand.

"I'm circling over to the inn," Lester said. "They'll put you up free if you need to stay till morning. I'll let them know you're coming."

Lester didn't want to go inside the hospital with Hugh, in case Charlie was dead.

Charlie wasn't dead. His head was wrapped in white bandages. His face was badly bruised, and one eye was swollen shut. He'd lost his two front teeth.

The nurse told Hugh the fog was to blame for Charlie's hitting the tree.

Hugh's bushy eyebrows lowered as he studied his son.

"Probably been drinking," Hugh said. "Would you like some coffee?" The nurse declined.

Lester came in. "If he's all right, I'm going home, then."

"He's banged up, that's all," Hugh told his neighbor. "I want to thank you for getting me here. Coffee?"

Lester said no to the offer.

After Lester left, the nurse returned and said they should turn out the lights in Charlie's room. She said she could bring in a chair, so Hugh could sit in the one that was already there and put his feet on the other.

"I think I'll get some sleep and come back in the morning," Hugh said. "Should be ready to get the Lizzie out of the woods by then."

Hugh exited the hospital drive. Netherland Inn Road was shrouded in river fog.

A coffeepot isn't much of a light when you're walking in the fog. Hugh could see his feet, and that was about the end of it. He was hit by a Model T and killed.

As a ghost, Hugh can see things better than when he was alive. He can see through the fog.

One night, he walked to a sharp bend in the road and, waving the enameled pot in his hand, signaled for an oncoming car to slow down. The driver saw Hugh's ghost and took his foot off the gas. The ghost disappeared in the fog.

The driver told his story the next day at a restaurant in Kingsport. Everyone there told everyone else.

When the night fog gathers thick as coffee on Netherland Inn Road, travelers coming upon a sharp curve see a man in overalls waving an enameled pot like he's signaling a train to stop. There hasn't been a wreck on that curve in decades.

FINAL CURTAIN
ORPHEUM THEATER,
203 SOUTH MAIN STREET,
MEMPHIS

GETTING TO THE HOSPITAL in a city turns out now and then to be the adventure of a lifetime. Sometimes, it's the final one.

The girl said to have been hit by the trolley on Beale Street in 1921 is called Mary by convenience. Her name was Beth. Still is.

And she wasn't hit by the trolley. She was bumped by a beige touring sedan when she darted across the street in front of the trolley. The man driving the car was badly shaken. He saw the flash of pigtails, felt the thump.

It wasn't his fault. He'd done nothing wrong. Yet it was his responsibility if the girl was injured.

Out of the car, the handsome driver with carefully combed hair helped Beth to her feet. One knobby knee was bloodied. Her dress was stained. A small cut was on her lip.

A crowd of curious onlookers gathered as the famous actor helped the girl into the passenger seat. He told those at the scene that he was taking the girl to the hospital.

Back in the driver's seat, he asked her name.

"Well, Beth, you look just fine to me, and I'm running late. How would you like a free seat in the theater? Have you ever been?"

Beth's mouth hurt a little, and her knee a little more. Something felt wrong in her stomach, like it was filling up with water. But she'd never been to the theater before.

"I'm late, you see. The audience is already in their seats," he explained,

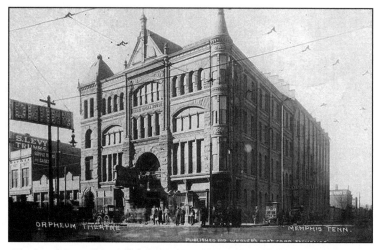

The Grand Opera, later called the Orpheum Theatre, in Memphis, Tennessee, is shown here in 1910 before it burned in 1923. It was replaced by the present Orpheum Theatre in 1928.

turning the beige sedan on to Main Street. "I'll take you to the hospital after."

"Will they let me in?"

"Of course they will," he assured her. "You're with me." He shot the girl a smile and a wink.

The gentleman smelled of lavender soap and talcum powder. Beth had never met a man who smelled like that. She felt completely grown up, just being in his car.

Back then, the Orpheum was the Grand Opera House. It was a five-floor theater, complete with balcony. The waterfall curtain on stage was maroon velvet. When the footlights came on, it looked blood-red.

Beth was given seat C-5 in the balcony, stage left. She watched the show in amazement. It was magnificent from the moment the curtain rose.

Eventually, Beth slumped in her seat. Her ears were ringing. Her stomach ached. By the time the final curtain fell, Beth was dead from internal injuries she'd suffered when the actor's car hit her square on.

Her body was taken to the hospital in an ambulance, after an usher discovered she wasn't moving, though her eyes were open. Beth died taking in the show. The look on her face was one of enchantment and surprise.

Now deceased, Beth quickly found her way back to her theater seat. She has experienced every show's final curtain since.

The Grand Opera House, which was razed by fire in 1923, was soon rebuilt as the Orpheum Theatre. Beth stayed put throughout it all.

Many people have claimed to see her ghost taking in the live productions at the Orpheum. And those claims are not to be taken lightly. Yul Brynner saw her when he performed here in *The King and I*. She's always in seat C-5 in the balcony. Actors on stage watch for her. Following the opening-night performance of *Fiddler on the Roof*, during which Beth's ghost was clearly visible, cast members held a séance in the balcony to see if there was anything they could do for her. Not knowing any better, they called her Mary.

To a Tennessee girl in pigtails, the theater must look like the inner dome of heaven. The Orpheum boasts elegant two-thousand-pound chandeliers. Gold leaf adorns the plaster relief over the stage.

For whatever reason, Beth's ghost is content to hold her seat at the Orpheum for eternity, it seems. She is known to run the aisles, bang doors backstage, and otherwise keep herself occupied during the day. So far, she hasn't spoken to anyone, though she is quick to move her feet out of the way for other theatergoers needing to find their seats on her row.

Beth may not talk to anyone because she doesn't know people are speaking to her. They're always talking to someone named Mary.

OTHER TENNESSEE SIGHTINGS

ANDERSONVILLE

A small, unincorporated community, Andersonville doesn't have a hospital. It does, however, have a hospital bed.

The bed on wheels that travels along Dark Hollow Road appears to serve as transport for a local ghost on his way to or from somewhere unknown. Local gossip suggests the hospital bed was the one an elderly gentleman used in his house during his final years, when he had in-home nursing care. The aged fellow fell in love with his nurse. Now dead, he is trying to find out where she lives.

The phantom hospital bed on Dark Hollow Road vanishes when traffic approaches. It then quickly reappears and keeps on going. The bed is also seen parked in front of homes early in the morning. It and its passenger vanish if someone tries to touch them.

"He'll find her one day," a resident said in a recent interview. "Then I suppose we won't be seeing that bed on Dark Hollow Road anymore."

CLARKSVILLE

Located just south of the Kentucky state line, Clarksville is a near neighbor of Fort Campbell. The Tennessee town of approximately fifty thousand people, settled in part by Continental Army soldiers after the Revolutionary War, has long been associated with the military.

The ghost of a man with no legs is seen as he walks by the doors of patient rooms on the first floor of Gateway Medical Center on Dunlop Lane in Clarksville. Some believe he is the ghost of a full-bodied man who has worn his legs away by walking in the afterlife.

FRANKLIN

Carnton Mansion saw service as a hospital during and after the Battle of Franklin. A cemetery near the two-story brick mansion is the final rest-

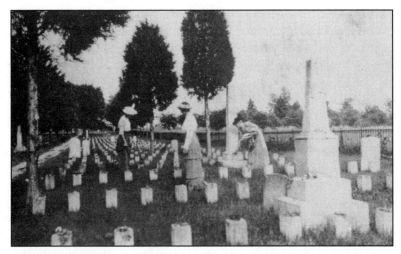

McGavock Confederate Cemetery near Carnton Mansion in Franklin, Tennessee, in 1890
Tennessee State Library & Archives

ing place of more than fifteen hundred Confederate soldiers. The bodies of four Southern generals who died of wounds suffered in the battle were displayed in state inside the mansion. To this day, the ghosts of fallen comrades rise from the cemetery and make their way to the mansion to pay their respects to the generals who lost their lives in the bloody battle.

FRANKLIN

A visually disturbing ghost haunts the outskirts of Franklin. The man attempts to hitch a ride by flapping an arm as he walks the highway past Pinkerton Park on his way out of town.

The ghostly hitchhiker appears to be a former patient of Confederate surgeon Deering J. Roberts, who established a field hospital in an old wagon shop in Franklin. Roberts vowed never to amputate a limb without the consent of the wounded. He recorded in his journal that one of his patients at the make-do hospital died after refusing amputation of a badly injured and infected arm. Deering noted that the soldier, who suffered from "nostalgia and despondency," had but one goal after being hospitalized, and that was to get up from his bed and walk home in time for Christmas. After repeated collapses while attempting to leave the hospital, the soldier succumbed on December 23, 1864.

Death will slow a person down, it's agreed. But dying doesn't necessarily mean a person stops trying.

KNOXVILLE

Dr. James Harvey Baker's antebellum house and clinic on Kingston Pike is now home to the Baker Peters Cigar and Literary Society and Jazz Club. Dr. Baker was killed by locally raised Union troops while treating wounded Confederate soldiers in his home. When Union troops raided the building one night, Dr. Baker barricaded himself in a room upstairs. Rather than troubling themselves to break down or remove the door, the Federals fired their weapons blindly through it and fatally shot the doctor, whose only crime was tending to the wounded in accordance with his professional oath.

Ghostly lantern lights appear in the middle of the night around the modern-day club on Kingston Pike. Soon afterward, guests sometimes hear the sound of muskets being fired.

KNOXVILLE

Hillcrest Health Care North, a nursing home on Beverly Park Circle, is closed now. Part of the old nursing home was a facility built as a tuberculosis hospital and sanatorium. The presence of asbestos makes the building unsafe for future use. Slated to be torn down once the money is raised, the stone structure is home to one of the happiest ghosts in the South. Said to be that of a maintenance man going about his work, he is heard early in the morning whistling a delightful tune.

MEMPHIS

Without saying a word, ghosts inside the former United States Marine Hospital, now the National Ornamental Metal Museum, make plenty of noise on a new stairway of the remodeled structure.

The brick building on a bluff overlooking the Mississippi River holds many secrets. Renovations that began in 1979 disturbed the nineteenth-century ghosts on the premises. Workers on hire from a nearby prison fled the basement and refused to return. Prison apparently was a friendlier place than the old hospital morgue.

A body chute into the morgue provided a handy means of moving deceased victims of a yellow-fever epidemic. The sealed-off chute, discovered during the renovations, was replaced with a fine set of stairs. Sadly, that didn't end the sound of bodies sliding into the basement morgue. Some days, they fall one after another. Standing at the bottom of the stairs, one can also hear the grunts and groans of those lifting the bodies and shoving them into the chute that is no longer there.

MORRISTOWN

Bethesda Church and Cemetery, a stop on the Tennessee Civil War Trail, served as a hospital and graveyard when Confederate general James Longstreet brought twenty-five thousand troops to the area in December 1863.

The brick building with two front doors was built in 1835. A tall ghost thought by many to have a pure white face walks through a closed door of the church early in the morning and continues to the graves. Without pause, he passes through headstones, trees, shrubs, and any people standing in the way. Visitors who catch a look at the six-foot-three apparition know why the face of this ghost of the Confederacy appears white. His head is wrapped in bandages.

Late in the evening, when the first stars appear, the ghost with a white face climbs out of his grave and walks back to the church, entering through the other door.

MOUNTAIN HOME

Appropriately nicknamed Bob by those who've seen him, the ghost of a World War I veteran wearing a doughboy helmet rises from a depression on the grounds of the James A. Quillen VA Medical Center in Mountain Home.

One patient there was a victim of shell shock, as it was called at the time, suffered during trench warfare. Believing he had come under enemy fire, the former soldier grabbed his helmet and headed to the duck pond on the grounds. Bob waded to the middle and lay down on the muddy bottom for protection. He drowned there.

The pond was drained but is still easily found. It appears as a distinct basin in an open field near the current administration building. Those with the patience of a fisherman will see a ghost helmet and face rise from the ground, look around, and quickly duck back into the grass. Bob's bob was a tactic of World War I soldiers, who needed to determine the location of opposing forces but had to be quick about it to keep from having their heads or helmets holed by rifle fire.

As a ghost at war, and as a rapidly appearing and disappearing target, Bob's done quite well all these years. He hasn't been shot yet.

ONEIDA

At midnight on May 23, 2012, the doors of the emergency room at Scott County Hospital were closed and locked. The hospital, shut down, was vacated and out of business. And there it sat, empty of all but ghosts, until December 2013, when it reopened as Pioneer Community Hospital. At that point, patients, staff, and visitors became reacquainted with Oneida's most famous ghost.

While a patient at Scott County Hospital, a young lady killed herself by taking a head-first dive from the foot of her bed and landing on her skull with enough force, and a large cracking sound, to do herself in. Although the patient took the dive on purpose, she may not have meant for it to be fatal. Either way, it was.

Her ghost now walks the new hospital, as it did the former one. She holds her arms out in front of her. Her skull is fissured at the forehead, and her neck is broken. According to all who've seen her, she makes a lasting impression, often being mistaken for a zombie.

PITTSBURG LANDING

The Battle of Shiloh, named for a small white church at the site, was fought in early April 1862. Union soldiers under General Ulysses S. Grant were camped on the west bank of the Tennessee River at Pittsburg Landing. Confederate forces under Generals Albert Sidney Johnston and P. G. T. Beauregard, thinking they'd had just about enough of Northern troops invading the South, launched a surprise attack on Grant. Their intention was to drive the Union troops away from the river and into a swamp, where the Yankees would be forced to surrender.

A fierce battle ensued. General Johnston was killed during the first day of fighting. Before it ended, the two-day Battle of Shiloh would become the costliest in American history to that time. Both sides suffered severe losses. More than three thousand men were killed and approximately fifteen thousand wounded. Union hospital boats steamed to the landing on the Tennessee River. Men in blue dashed in pairs, carrying stretchers to transport Union wounded to the vessels, where teams of surgeons waited with their saws.

On rare occasions, the Union orderlies reappear as ghosts, always in pairs. One man runs six feet or so behind the other. The ghostly figures emerge from the Tennessee and eventually return to the river's edge and—while onlookers gawk—disappear.

TEXAS

KICKS
OLD BAPTIST ST. ANTHONY'S HOSPICE HOSPITAL,
NEAR INTERSTATE 40,
AMARILLO

HUMANS POSSESS FAR MORE than the basic five senses talked about in school.

One of the most pronounced is a sense of safety and, conversely, the oppressive sense that something is wrong. This important sense accounts for the willies, the jitters, and hair lifting at the back of one's neck. Everyone has experienced the sense that something's just not right. And the sense of being watched when no one is there.

It is by means of their sixth sense, seventh sense, or eighth or ninth sense that many people first experience a ghost. Some find it difficult to admit they had a ghost experience. Others say they felt a presence or that they knew, just knew, someone was there when there was otherwise nothing to see, hear, touch, or smell—no actual physical evidence of a ghost.

Yet the ghost was real.

Could be, plain old fear is a sense more people should pay attention to. Humans fear hospitals. They are places where even visitors don't want to stay too long. It's in the gut, in the bones, and on the surface of the skin. Heaven forbid you're admitted as a patient.

Every patient's hope is not to be in the hospital long. It smells like a hospital, for one thing. And the staff is always sticking needles in you, or inserting catheters, for some reason or another. Does hospital food need to be mentioned?

And people die there. Most of those people are patients.

Hospital treatment for injury or illness, surgery to make a repair or remove a little this or that—most of us go through such experiences at one time or another. Maybe just a quick shot for pain, a setting of a broken nose, or a few stitches to close a cut.

Other patients, however, are not so lucky. They find themselves admitted to a hospital for the remainder of life. This is the case for terminal patients admitted to Baptist St. Anthony's Hospice Hospital in Amarillo, Texas, an institution with an exceptional reputation for compassionate care. Patients come to BSA Hospice Hospital to stay. Period. Although one or two might be looking for a way out after their deaths.

When the hospital recently moved to new facilities, the old BSA Hospice Hospital—not far from I-40, the original Route 66—was closed. And the ghost of a patient at the old hospital decided not to take death lying down. He managed to get himself into a wheelchair and roll outdoors into the parking lot. Wearing an open-back hospital gown and a rather extreme case of bed hair, he kept rolling.

No tubes, no needles. The ghost made the most of it.

An Amarillo couple was walking by the old hospital, holding hands, when they saw a man in a wheelchair exiting the building. The doors were locked, but there he was on the sidewalk. Then he rolled into the parking lot. The wife remembered that his rather long, white hair stuck straight out from one side of his head, as if it had been plastered there.

"He started screaming, and he rolled right into the middle of the road, in the middle of oncoming traffic," she said. "Nobody else saw that he was there, just my husband and me. Then, all of a sudden, he vanished."

Vanished, or turned the corner? The ramp to old Route 66 was only a few blocks away. Drivers and passengers in the eastbound lanes are advised to be on the lookout.

THE WAY OUT
OLD MERCY HOSPITAL,
1500 LOGAN STREET,
LAREDO

THE IDEA OF A GHOST using a messenger from nature is well established throughout the South. Birds, butterflies, dogs, and even foxes are commonly believed to carry messages from recently deceased loved ones. They usually appear soon after a funeral and hang around a few days to be sure they are noticed.

Sometimes, they appear shortly before a funeral and alert people to the fact that someone is dying. As with England's famous black hound, known to lurk outside a house when someone is soon to be in mortal danger, a messenger animal is a harbinger. Hounds that howl on moonless nights when someone in the house has died remind us that animals are in close contact with the spirit world. In the Deep South, including parts of Texas, dearly departed loved ones often show up as white dogs at night. They usually have a direct message for family members who encounter them.

Ghosts are often messengers from beyond life, their singular goal being to get messages across to those from our world. In the case of one such ghost, a hospital nun in Laredo, actions speak louder than words.

The Sisters of Mercy arrived in South Texas in 1875. The order established Laredo's first hospital, a twelve-bed facility, in 1894. Until recently, the Sisters of Mercy provided service to the community at a large medical complex on Logan Street. Closed and offered for sale in 2013, the facility is now vacant.

Well, mostly vacant. The ghost of Sister Mary Elizabeth Ryan hasn't yet found her way to the new Laredo Medical Center on Saunders Street. She may not want to. She's more concerned with people finding their way to the afterlife. A dedicated servant to the sick and dying, the ghost of

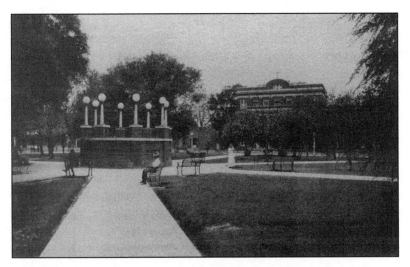

Postcard of Jarvis Plaza in Laredo, Texas. Mercy Hospital is visible in the background, early 20th century.
LAREDO PUBLIC LIBRARY, LAREDO, TEXAS

Sister Mary Elizabeth knows where people go when they're dead. She's been there often enough. She's there now.

Sister Mary Elizabeth was first noticed as a ghost in the old Mercy Hospital in 1991, when a visitor who exited on the wrong floor became lost. The visitor believed she may have exited into the basement. She walked back and forth along the hallways, searching for the place she meant to go. She obviously looked lost.

"A nun came out of nowhere," she said. "I asked if there was a way out, and she pointed to a door."

The visitor thanked her and pushed open the door to what turned out to be the hospital morgue.

When she turned back to question her benefactor, "she was gone. The nun never spoke a word."

The ghost of Sister Mary Elizabeth never does, people have learned.

Sometimes, when she's in a hurry to reach a person, she barks to announce that she's coming.

The old hospital is a large, multi-floor facility. When the ghost is far away from where visitors appear lost, it comes to their assistance on four legs. A dog with a silky black coat and a collar of pure white fur swiftly approaches in a dead run through the hospital hallways. Once the dog is near, it stands on its hind legs and becomes the full-bodied ghost of Sister Mary Elizabeth. Making steady, if slower, progress, the nun then walks the lost visitors to the morgue. Her message, of course, is letting them know the way out—the way out of this life and into the next.

Ask not for whom the stainless-steel gurney rolls. And don't bother asking Sister Mary Elizabeth anything. All she'll do is point.

SOMETHING TO REMEMBER
EMILY MORGAN HOTEL,
705 EAST HOUSTON STREET,
SAN ANTONIO

MANY PEOPLE THINK of the Alamo only as the location of a siege and battle in 1836. They consider the mission little more than a fort temporarily occupied by early Texans in the war with Mexico. But the Alamo has a much richer tradition. And like all early missions, it provided hospital care to the local population. One victim from those distant years may still be around today.

Missions were established to introduce members of the native population to an entirely new way of life. Begun in 1718 by a group of Franciscan monks who constructed a small chapel at San Antonio de Valero, the original mission that became the Alamo was also a school, a farm, a livestock ranch, a food-storage site, a hospital, and a graveyard. The Alamo provided a place of worship and a fortification for the conversion of indigenous people.

In 1739, the mission grounds saw the construction of a large thatch-topped hospital with a small adobe hut on one end. Those were the days of smallpox, the Red Plague. As the number of victims increased, the thatched roof was extended on wooden posts impaled in the sun-parched soil.

Prior to General Santa Anna's 1836 victory, an important turning point in Texas history, countless bodies were buried on the wide-spread grounds of the mission. Many of those bodies are under the modern buildings that now surround the Alamo.

Originally, the mission did not record the number of burials outside the churchyard. Church records, however, do exist. Priests from the mission had conducted the formal burials of 465 people by 1749. Records kept by priests from 1749 to 1782 indicate an additional 489 burials. The locations of most of those graves are unknown. Many informal burials of the unconverted were attended to by family members and were not recorded by the priests.

The Red Plague was a most unpleasant way to die. It was also ugly. Although the infection initially appeared as a rash of tiny pimples on the lining of the throat and mouth, victims of the smallpox plague were soon covered with a blossoming of fluid-filled red blisters resembling roses. Within days, the fluid in the blisters was replaced with dead flesh. Then things worsened.

The active lesions were excruciatingly painful. Providing comfort to those dying of the pox required the compassion of a saint. The available treatment in 1739 consisted of cool water, the repeated application of a damp cloth, and a quick burial.

The elaborate Medical Arts Building was erected in the 1920s across the street from the Alamo, on ground that had served as the mission's hospital during the smallpox epidemic. Now the Emily Morgan Hotel, the V-shaped building served a number of years as the city's downtown hospital and provided additional clinic space for several privately owned practices.

The structure is centered by a castle tower. A row of spire-topped windows extends to either side on the top floor. A remarkable example of urban Gothic Revival architecture, the building is one of San Antonio's most recognizable landmarks. Unique gargoyles, fashioned as people suffering from a variety of ailments, are haunting details of the exterior.

Guests in the hotel have reported a large number of ghost encounters. One frequent sighting occurs on the eleventh floor. An old woman in a hospital gown walks the hallway, pausing to weep before vanishing at the end of the hall.

The most interesting ghost, however, is a rather pleasant young girl who hums and sings in the hallways. Hearing her sing is the way most guests experience the girl's presence. On other occasions, she enters the

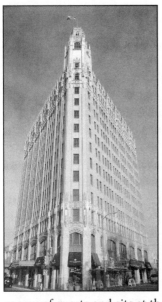

The Emily Morgan Hotel in San Antonio, Texas
DAVID R. TRIBBLE

rooms of guests and sits at the foot of their beds. There, she materializes into a full apparition. Sometimes, she asks, in an eager burst of Spanish, if the hotel guest would like to sing along. The temperature in the room drops dramatically when she is present. It is speculated that the girl with long, dark hair and dark eyes has returned from her grave to visit a friend or relative who died in the hospital.

Those who pay careful attention realize the girl is blind. Blindness was a common result of smallpox among those few who, long before a vaccination was developed, survived the Red Plague. This suggests her ghost may have been present at the location more than a hundred years prior to the construction of the building that houses the hotel.

The Emily Morgan Hotel is listed on the National Register of Historic Places as part of Alamo Plaza. The listing doesn't mention the ghosts or the smallpox plague of 1739. It also doesn't mention the fact that people on the city sidewalks surrounding the Alamo are walking on dead people—dead people no one remembers.

OTHER TEXAS SIGHTINGS

ATHENS

Henderson County Memorial Hospital, built in 1948 and closed in 1982 upon the completion of East Texas Medical Center, has stood abandoned for more than thirty years. The ghosts there need someone to talk to. Especially receptive to communication through a Ouija board, one ghost enjoys answering questions about being dead. He identifies himself as Mark by spelling out his name on the board. Apparently, the afterlife is filled with all manner of problems for Mark. He complains endlessly. People, he says, have no respect for the dead. And the building could use some heat. He also wants to know why it has no electricity. He can't play the radio or watch television. As for having running water, Mark gave up on that years ago.

The county paid more than a hundred thousand dollars to have asbestos removed from the structure in 2007, a prerequisite to demolition. Yet the building was saved and is currently undergoing conversion to an assisted-living facility for veterans. Mark will soon have new people to talk to—people who don't get up and leave after an hour or two.

CORSICANA

Some ghosts have no expiration date. They live in the shadows.

Although the old Navarro Hospital in Corsicana has been torn down, a ghost continues to make his home there. He's usually at the top of the old steps to the building. The steps are all that remain of the demolished structure on Hospital Drive. Well, steps and a tree, neither of which has provided the ghost with a stairway to heaven.

The ghost sits waiting on the steps during the day and climbs into the tree next to them at night. He is most easily seen in the evening. When a car parks in front of the steps, the ghost climbs out of his tree as a shadow in darkness. He approaches the car by descending the steps, becoming more clearly visible as he nears. At the bottom step, he is a fully visible apparition of a man.

By honking the horn, visitors find the ghost rapidly returns to a shadow of his former self and climbs back up the steps to his tree.

DALLAS

The old Parkland Hospital on Maple Drive has been closed for years. Recently renovated for other uses, the building is haunted by a horse-drawn ambulance. Without a rider in the top seat, it pulls up in front and waits. When someone approaches from inside the building, the horse and wagon disappear, and the resounding plod of hooves fades into the distance.

From force of habit, the ghost horse brings the ambulance wagon, apparently unoccupied, to the front of the hospital from the afterlife.

EL PASO

Providence Memorial Hospital, on the eastern edge of the University of Texas at El Paso, is home to a devoted head nurse who continues to check in on patients long after her death. An example of a ghost who won't stop doing in death what she was doing at the end of her life, Bertha appears in patient rooms, smiles at the occupants, and leaves. Soon afterward, a staff nurse arrives.

Bertha, it appears, likes to get there first.

GALVESTON

Some old sailors return to water after they die.

The old United States Marine Hospital, built in 1931, has been converted into a modern apartment complex. Of the forty-eight units, one includes the hospital room where a former sailor died. His ghost seems to be trapped inside the building. But that doesn't keep him from returning to the sea. Or at least as close as he can get. This ghost sings in the shower. There, water running or not, he has been heard to sing for hours. He's particularly fond of belting out an old Howard Dietz song, "Alone

Together." The title pretty much sums up the experience of being the only dead person in the apartment.

HOUSTON

Death marked the spot where the old Jefferson Davis Hospital was erected. Built in 1924, the hospital sat atop land that was once Houston City Cemetery. The city owned the land and believed it could do what it wanted with it. But Houston had a problem. After years of protest, the graves of thirty-two Confederate veterans were restored and properly marked.

Other underground occupants were not as fortunate. One such group was the city-buried victims of an 1840s yellow-fever epidemic. During excavation work to replace old utility lines, approximately sixty "black-earth graves" were uncovered. The unmarked graves had two common characteristics: the bodies were laid facing west and were buried without coffins. The remains, wrapped in cloth at the time of internment, were stained with dirt when discovered.

Not having coffins allowed for easy escape for the ghosts of the dead. They moved inside the handsome red-brick hospital built atop their graves. The oft-spotted, mud-spattered apparitions became known as "the ghosts with dirty faces."

Closed in 1938, the hospital sat empty of all but ghosts for decades. Eventually renovated, the building reopened in 2005 as the Elder Street Artists Loft. Current occupants continue to report ghosts with dirt on their faces—although there is some difficulty in distinguishing them from the artists who work in the loft studios.

LUBBOCK

Apparently, it's hard to get to heaven from Lubbock.

A dying patient quartered in the original West Texas Sanitarium near Avenue L and Broadway tried to escape his unhappy fate on earth by chiseling a hole in the wall with a fork. Using his hands, he enlarged the opening until it was large enough to crawl inside.

He died in the wall. Once his body was retrieved, his ghost stayed where it was, perhaps figuring the hole in the wall was his only path to heaven, or his only means of avoiding a more downwardly destination.

When the sanitarium was razed, the ghost moved inside the walls of the Methodist church nearby. The ghost most often manifests himself as fingers pushing out from the walls, as if to test their durability. At other times, the contours of his face press out from the sheetrock. The ghost quickly goes away when noticed.

A fear of one's destiny in the afterlife is sufficient motivation to keep some ghosts from leaving their earthly bonds.

MISSION

A number of ghosts sit perfectly still in the Mission Regional Medical Center emergency room. Each apparition is of an injured man or woman. Two are children. Their main goal appears to be not to disturb anyone. Research suggests the ghosts are not of people who died at the same time, which may indicate a recruiter ghost among the dead. Through example, a recruiter ghost encourages other ghosts to do the same thing he or she is doing. The remaining ghosts are followers.

At Mission Regional, the additional ghosts are followers in more ways than one. If a living person in the emergency room accidentally looks one of them in the eye, that ghost becomes theirs. The ghost goes along with them when they leave. Also called "come-along ghosts," followers attach themselves to their companions' lives, sitting quietly in their houses, the backseat of their cars, or beside them on a bench at the mall. Wherever the humans go, they have their ghosts right there.

The only way to be rid of the presence is to return to the hospital, take a seat in the emergency room, and wait for the follower ghost to reappear. Then the human must tell it in no uncertain terms to stay, and do so without looking into its eyes.

PALESTINE

The former Palestine Memorial Hospital on East Brazos Street looks so much like a sprawling hotel that you'd expect to find an ice machine on every floor. But the abandoned facility is not a place you'd like to stay. The city morgue was in the basement, and no one leaves the lights on for you. The basement is where one of the hospital's remaining ghosts hangs out. Or maybe it would be more correct to say hangs "up." The female ghost levitates, floating to the ceiling, where she quickly disappears. Every time she has been seen thus far, she ends up stuck overhead. Even in the afterlife, ceilings evidently have a way of blocking one's path.

PAMPA

Not much is going on inside the abandoned, three-story Worley Hospital in Pampa, Texas. That is, until you go into the basement. There, the incinerator door makes a noise when opened, as you might expect an iron door to do. What you don't expect is that instead of a harsh squeak, the door's opening releases the scream of a woman. The scream is loud enough to light up the darkness. She is said to continue screaming until the door of the incinerator is once again closed.

SAN ANTONIO

Known locally as "the insane asylum," San Antonio State Hospital was built in the late 1880s. The abandoned buildings out on Farm Road were recently demolished. Some ghosts, it is believed, were bulldozed underground inside lidded jars. The jars stored brain tissue from patients who died at the asylum during a period when studying the brains of the mentally disturbed was a popular method of scientific inquiry. Numbered labels lacking the patients' names but noting their age and body weight at the time of death were affixed to the specimen jars. The pieces of brain matter, submerged in a liquid preservative, were never actually studied. They were stored on shelves in a corner of the basement, along with broken bits of the old building and its furnishings. Not quite a happy bunch, those brains.

The jars may contain ghosts along with the cerebral tissue. Many jars have broken underground, their contents leeched into the soil. Others likely remain intact. Either way, the ghosts who haunt the location don't actually inhabit the jars. The hauntings are brainless dead searching for their thoughts. The ghosts roam the bulldozed fields at night, always during a full moon, hoping to relocate their brains. They stare vacantly at the ground and walk in ever-widening circles.

Local residents are fearful of the wandering apparitions. It is believed that people who walk or drive into the path of the brain seekers will end up missing a few thoughts of their own.

For these ghosts, any brains they can get their hands on—including yours—might just do.

TAYLOR

Wedemeyer Hospital and Sanitarium, established in 1915, sits far back from the road on Seventh Street. Private residences are to either side. The historic structure, now undergoing renovation, boasts six white columns supporting a second-story gallery in front. The long driveway from Seventh passes through a porte-cochère attached to the left side of the hospital. The roof of the porte-cochère was originally accessed from the upper level of the structure, also known as Taylor Hospital.

The driveway to the side of the building is where the most active ghost in Taylor begins, and continues, his haunt. The former resident, who suffered from acute alcoholism, loved to drive. Once hospitalized, the gentleman was no longer allowed access to a car. In fact, he wasn't allowed out of the building, other than to stroll the roof of the porte-cochère.

As his liver began to fail, he made plans to take a spin around town. One night, he climbed down from the rooftop and borrowed Dr. George Wedemeyer's sleek sedan. But before he could pilot the vehicle on to Seventh Street, he died, his hands clutching the wheel as the car idled, its nose not quite making it into the street.

Staff members carried his body inside. But his ghost walked onto the rooftop, thinking it would be better to position himself on that spot in the afterlife than anywhere else.

Today, cars left in the driveway find themselves driven by a ghost to the edge of the street—but no farther. One living driver who located his vehicle stalled at the street end of the driveway saw a pair of hands clutching the steering wheel.

The car-thief ghost of Taylor, Texas, knows where he's going. He just never gets too far.

VICTORIA

Levi was driving with his dog in his truck one night in Victoria. The happy duo was making its way to a favorite fishing spot just off the interstate near the bridge over the Guadalupe River. In South Texas, the big ones bite at night. But not that night. Levi and his faithful companion eventually returned to the truck empty-handed.

As they got in, Levi thought he heard a guy moaning.

"My dog was going crazy," he said. "She started barking and flying around in circles."

Someone was tapping the outside of the passenger window.

"I got out with my pistol drawn," Levi reported, "and there I saw a boy of fifteen or sixteen."

Levi described the youth as having long hair, frightened eyes, and blood on his shirt. He was very pale. As pale as a ghost.

"He was begging for a ride to get medical help. I walked toward the boy to help him, and he disappeared."

When Levi got back in the driver's seat, he felt the presence of someone else in the cab.

"My dog was sitting there as if she were being petted," he said.

While Levi hadn't caught any fish, it looked like he had snagged a ghost.

He drove to DeTar Hospital North and pulled to a stop in the parking lot near the emergency room. He realized only then that there was nothing he could really do to get help for an injured boy who wasn't physically there. Levi walked around to the passenger door and opened it. The ghost moved through Levi as a cold mass of air and was gone.

No one is sure where the boy died. Or when. His ghost, though, is in the parking lot of DeTar North on Medical Drive in Victoria.

WICHITA FALLS

At North Texas State Hospital, several shadows of people who aren't there join office workers for lunch in the current administration center.

The building originally housed patients. The ghosts are shades. A shade is a particular and peculiar type of ghost that casts a shadow without ever being seen. The bodiless spirit then inhabits the shadow, which moves about on its own.

At North Texas State Hospital, an instigator shade seems to have taught other ghosts the trick. What one spirit does to exist after death, other dead in the vicinity may copy.

VIRGINIA

HEART THROB
SENTARA VIRGINIA BEACH GENERAL HOSPITAL, 1060 FIRST COLONIAL ROAD, VIRGINIA BEACH

RACHEL DROVE HER CAR into the crowded lot near the emergency-room entrance to Sentara Virginia Beach General Hospital. She was there to pick up her boyfriend, who worked as a nurse. It was getting dark.

She found a spot under the trees at the edge of the lot. Rachel pulled in and switched on her flashers so he could locate the car quickly. She wasn't allowed to call him on his cell when he was working, so she texted a quick message.

"Soon? Under the trees in the front lot."

He texted back a few minutes later.

"Soon! Sorry. :("

It wasn't cold, but the ocean breeze was chilly. Rachel kept her windows up. She soon was lost in her thoughts. She planned what she and her boyfriend would do if they missed their reservation at the restaurant. They'd probably sit at the bar and drink, she thought. Eat hot wings or bar tacos. He'd drink too much, and she wouldn't because one of them had to drive. He'd tell bad jokes all night. When they got to his place, he'd want her to stay. She wouldn't. It was no big deal. She'd had worse nights.

That's when she saw the shadow come down from the trees. Rachel tilted her head and squinted to see it better. It must have been a trick of the headlights from cars passing on First Colonial Road. She waited for a repeat performance. Instead, the shadow darted toward her car.

She texted her boyfriend again, just to keep from feeling alone. And vulnerable.

"Reservations."

The shadow moved closer. Rachel saw a glint of light in the middle of the gossamer apparition. As the shadow neared, the glinting object turned out to be the business end of a stethoscope the ghost wore around its neck.

Puzzled and mesmerized by the appearance of a shadowy ghost in the parking lot, Rachel watched and waited. She wouldn't scream or start honking her horn or anything crazy, she decided. She was thirty-two years old, not some little kid.

That's when two things happened at once. The circular piece of the stethoscope pressed flat against the windshield, and she felt a cold sensation on the left side of her chest. Rachel gasped. The stethoscope moved across the glass in a small arc. The cold spot Rachel felt moved with it, only soon it was warm instead of cold.

When the piece of round metal stopped, Rachel could hear her heartbeat as loud as thunder. The sound of it filled the car. Her pulse raced. Rachel closed her eyes tight to keep from screaming. Then, out of breath, she laid on the horn.

The stethoscope disappeared. Her boyfriend rapped on the passenger window. Rachel nearly jumped out of her skin. The shadow, she noticed, was moving back into the trees. She pressed the button to unlock the door.

"Sorry I'm late," he said, getting in. "You don't have to get all honky about it."

Rachel smiled as best she could. Her forehead was beaded with sweat. The sound of her heartbeat faded, but it was still there, pounding in her ears.

"Want to hear something funny?" he asked. "Just before I left, I put the stethoscope on this woman. She was yammering away, and I couldn't hear a heartbeat. Turns out she was dead. But I swear she kept talking."

"Dead?"

"Dead as dust," he told her.

"Who was it?" Rachel wanted to know.

"Some dead doctor came by to get her blood pressure. I swear she was talking after she died. No joke. Can you believe it?"

"Yes," Rachel said, thinking the dead doctor was the shadow that had approached her car.

"Here's the other thing. The doctor was wearing a lab coat and a nametag. And the name was the same as that doctor who died, like, ten years ago."

"What did you do?"

"Well, after I checked the woman's name at the desk, she was gone. I didn't stick around to look for her. I knew you were waiting. One of the other nurses said she was a ghost. That's when I realized my stethoscope was missing."

Rachel breathed in deeply and slowly let it out. As she drove out of the parking lot, she smiled at the trees. *Nice work*, she thought.

Her heartbeat was normal. And she knew where to find her boyfriend's stethoscope. Rachel decided not to tell him. He had a degree in nursing and wouldn't believe that sort of thing.

"What do you think really happened?" she asked once they were on First Colonial.

"Prank," he said, shrugging. "You?"

"I think sometimes people mistake emergency flashers as a signal that you need help," Rachel said.

"Where did that come from?" He laughed.

"The trees," she replied.

A MISSING HOSPITAL TRAIN
COHOKE CROSSROADS,
WEST POINT

THE RICHMOND AND YORK RIVER RAILROAD, providing vital passage into and out of the capital of the Confederacy, was routinely sabotaged by Union forces during the War Between the States. One such act of sabotage resulted in a derailment approaching Cohoke Crossroads in rural West Point, Virginia.

Soldiers recently wounded in battle were on their way to the hospitals in Richmond. A steam engine pulling a single hospital car on a hastily arranged late-night run went off the tracks where the iron rails had been torn loose and removed by saboteurs. All aboard died when the car left the tracks, overturned, and plunged into a ravine. Since the soldiers were the most severely wounded among their comrades, they had a small chance of survival even had the hospital car not derailed.

The attendant surgeons and two railway workers, now dead with the others, decided their duty was not complete. Their ghosts joined those of the maimed and weary soldiers, most of whom were amputees. Together, they formed a line on the tracks. Instead of going to the hospitals, they would return to battle. In the front, one of the surgeons carried a salvaged railway lantern. Another that burned less brightly was carried at the rear of the line. Soldiers who were not ambulatory in life found they could walk as ghosts. Following the railroad tracks, they began their march to provide needed reinforcement of the Confederate lines.

Their return to battle has become a march that never ends. The ghosts do not reach their destination but rather dissipate into the afterlife somewhere along the line.

That doesn't mean they've given up. The line of dead set out on their long walk over and over again, almost nightly, always beginning at the time of the derailment. They're needed somewhere, and they mean to get there.

Today, the lantern light—and only the light—can be seen by those who come upon the ghost march at Cohoke Crossroads. Onlookers take positions where the tracks cross the road and wait. The light appears in the distance, only to grow brighter as the ghosts approach. Still following the rails, the lantern crosses the road and goes out some distance ahead.

"I went to the site with my mom and dad and some other adults," noted Tim Fry, now a captain of ocean rescue in southern Florida. "They parked on the tracks with two cars bumper to bumper. The light appeared and disappeared several times."

Tim recalled seeing the light go over the car hoods and continue down the tracks. "My father never believed the story until he saw the light that night."

Tim's mother, Mary Ann, is a retired nurse. She has seen the light on at least six occasions, but also recalls being present on nights when it did not appear.

"The light is round," she recently said. She described how it came forward along, and somewhat above, the railroad tracks. "There did not seem to be any beam of light, just a round glow." The ghost lantern slowly advanced. "It came toward us, then disappeared," she said. "Or so we thought. When we turned around, we saw the light had passed and was going down the tracks away from us."

Others over the years have parked cars across the tracks in an attempt to block the light from moving on. But it has always continued, although there are reports of unexplained handprints on cars after the light is gone.

West Point is a popular site with ghost hunters. One favored location for viewing the light is now on private land and should not be visited without permission. The rails were recently removed at that spot.

WITCH GHOST
LYNNHAVEN RIVER AT THE END OF DUCKING POINT TRAIL, VIRGINIA BEACH

THE GHOST OF GRACE WHITE SHERWOOD, a midwife, haunts the banks of the Lynnhaven River, where she was dunked, tied thumb to toe, while being tried for witchcraft in 1706.

Midwifery was a common and useful health-care service in colonial America, at a time when what few hospitals there were could not be bothered with assisting women in childbirth. A combination pharmacologist and obstetrician, a midwife was a knowledgeable herbalist and healer. As well as administering herbal teas to relieve cramps, headaches, and sleeplessness, a midwife also treated injuries, especially cuts and burns. She knew how to stem bleeding. And more than a few midwives knew how to set broken bones.

In short, midwives were lay doctors. Since they had healing powers at their beckoning, however, they were often accused of sorcery and witchcraft, especially when things went wrong. No good deed goes unpunished.

After a neighbor, Elizabeth Hill, miscarried, she publicly blamed Sherwood for "bewitchment." Already having faced such charges—including those of transforming herself into a cat, damaging crops, and causing the death of livestock—Sherwood was taken to trial on the new accusation, thereby becoming the last person in Virginia tried for witchcraft.

When taken inside the parish church and ordered to ask forgiveness for witchery, Sherwood replied, "I be not a witch. I be a healer."

The justices of Princess Anne County impaneled a jury, made up of women, and ordered them to act as fact-finders by searching Sherwood's

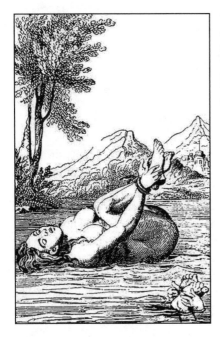

This 17th-century engraving depicts a "ducking" or dunking ordeal similar to the one given to Grace White Sherwood as part of her trial for witchcraft in 1706.
WETHERSFIELD HISTORICAL SOCIETY

home for "waxen or baked figures" that would prove she was a witch. The citizen jury proved one thing only—that they were wiser than the justices. They refused to conduct the search.

Another jury of "ancient and knowing women" was soon appointed. The old ladies were charged to look for markings on Sherwood's body that might be brands of the devil. They discovered two "marks not like theirs or like those of any other woman." The forewoman of this jury was Elizabeth Barnes, who in 1698 had accused Sherwood of assuming the form of a black cat, entering Barnes's home through a keyhole, jumping onto Elizabeth's bed, and whipping her. It was apparently easier to claim that a cat came through a keyhole and did you damage than it was to confess that your husband beat you.

The overseeing colonial authorities in Williamsburg, unwilling to declare Sherwood a witch on the word of Elizabeth Barnes, instructed the local court to examine the case more fully. The sheriff of Princess Anne County subsequently took Sherwood into custody. Maximilian Boush, a warden of Lynnhaven Parish Church, acted as prosecutor. A trial by ducking, a colonial term for dunking, was ordered.

In July 1706, Sherwood was taken to the edge of the Lynnhaven River, where she would be tossed from a boat into the water. The principles of trial by water were such that if Sherwood floated, she would be proven guilty of witchcraft. If she sank, she was innocent.

Sherwood was undressed by five women from the parish church, who examined her body for any devices she might use to free herself. Sherwood was then covered with a sack. The six justices who had ordered the trial by ducking rowed into the river in one boat. The sheriff, the prosecutor, and Sherwood set out in another.

Two hundred yards from shore, Sherwood was bound hand to foot, as was required for a legal ducking. Her right thumb was tied to her left big toe, and her left thumb to her right big toe. Thereupon, she was cast into the river.

The midwife and herbal healer quickly floated to the surface. Giving her one last chance to prove her innocence, the sheriff tied a thirteen-pound Bible around Sherwood's neck. This time, she sank, but the Bible became untied and Sherwood returned to the surface, guilty as the devil. She was a witch. It had been proven in "court." The final trial in America for practicing witchcraft was over.

Rather than being put to death, as witches had in Salem, Massachusetts, Sherwood was sentenced to jail, where she was held until 1714. That year, she is recorded to have paid taxes on her 145-acre property, which Virginia's lieutenant governor helped her recover from Princess Anne County. The midwife is thought to have lived the remainder of her life quietly until her recorded death in 1740. Her will noted that Sherwood, in the year of her death, was a widow.

Her ghost returns to the place of her ducking. Once a year, on a sunny day in July, a thoroughly soaked page of an ancient Bible floats to the surface of Lynnhaven River and makes its way to shore. Residents note that the page can be seen shining, brightly reflecting the sunlight.

Virginia Beach residents want you to know that they feel badly about Sherwood's having been tried as a witch in such a barbaric manner. A local midwife didn't deserve to be treated like that in their community.

A bronze statue of Grace White Sherwood holding a basket of rosemary, a raccoon at her side, was placed in 2007 on the site of Sentara Bayside Hospital, close to the locations of both the colonial courthouse and the ducking point. The raccoon is said to represent Sherwood's love of animals, and the rosemary her knowledge of herbal healing.

A local legend in Virginia Beach is that all the rosemary growing there came from a single plant Sherwood carried in an eggshell from England.

Really? Sounds about as reasonable as tying a woman's thumbs to her toes and tossing her into a lake to see if she's a witch.

STINKY MAN
CHIMBORAZO MEDICAL MUSEUM, 3215 EAST BROAD STREET, RICHMOND

IT WAS ALREADY DARK when Carlton Reed pulled his car alongside the curb. He leaned out the window.

"Let's go for a ride somewhere," he said.

"Maybe, but I have to be back at Linda's by ten o'clock. That's when her mother gets home."

Peggy's mom was strict. The sixteen-year-old was spending the night with Linda, or Peggy wouldn't be out at all.

"Yeah, sure."

"Promise?"

Carlton crossed his finger over the left pocket of his shirt.

"Get in," he said.

Luckily, Peggy was wearing her cutest top and her best shoes for autumn. Her jeans fit like a glove. She only wished she'd put on lipstick and perfume.

She was flattered the senior was interested in being with her. Carlton was popular in school. He ran with a cool crowd, to which neither she nor Linda belonged. If Peggy played her cards right, he might take her to some of the cool parties in private homes that year. Or maybe he'd ask her to prom. From the looks of things, he liked her. And she decided to like him back.

They stopped for frozen yogurt. Carlton paid for hers. No one was there who Peggy knew, which was a shame.

"Ten o'clock," Peggy reminded him. She wished he'd hold her hand.

Back in the car, Carlton made his way out of the Northside District and crossed on to Broad Street in the old part of town.

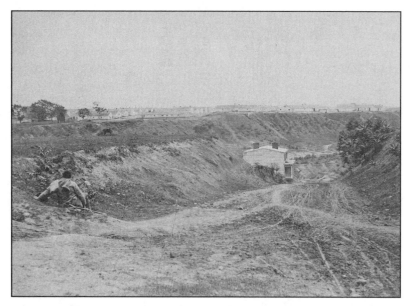

The Chimborazo Hospital, called the "hospital on the hill," pictured here in 1865. It is now the site of the Chimborazo Medical Museum in Richmond, Virginia. LIBRARY OF CONGRESS, PRINTS AND PHOTOGRAPHS DIVISION, LC-DIG-PPMSCA-33629

"I know a place where we can talk," he said.

"Talk about what?" she asked.

"Your lips," he said. "Your crazy, kissable lips."

She smiled. Peggy liked him, the way you like a song you already know the words to.

Carlton drove with his arm out the window. He made his way on to East Grace Street. Looking for the two trees that marked the driveway to a fenced-off lot and blocked the streetlight, Carlton was startled to see a slumped figure staggering along the road. The man was clutching his stomach with both hands.

"Stop," Peggy said. "He needs help."

Before Carlton came alongside the strange nighttime figure, a disgusting odor filled the car. The olfactory assault was not lost on Peggy. She clamped her hand over her mouth and nose. Carlton came to a stop. He rolled his window halfway up.

"Need help?" he said from the side of his mouth, turning his face away from, rather than toward, the window.

"Hospital," the man said clearly.

He removed one hand from low on his stomach and pointed in the direction of the old Chimborazo site at the top of Hospital Hill. The deeply etched expression on the man's face spoke of the distress he was in, as did the smell. Carlton couldn't leave him. Peggy curled sideways in her seat and stuck her head out the passenger window for air.

The odor was thick and dangerous. It smelled like diarrhea and rotted meat.

"Get in," Carlton said between clenched teeth. He popped open the door locks.

The stumbling figure obliged. But instead of opening the door, he climbed onto the trunk of the car, where he placed his feet on the rear bumper and bent forward in pain until his head nearly touched his knees.

As Carlton drove slowly away, he rolled his window all the way down. He coughed. The smell was that of illness and death.

Although the ghost hadn't said specifically, Carlton knew exactly where he wanted to go. His older brother had talked about Stinky Man before. Carlton had always believed the story was some sort of urban legend. The smell in his car said otherwise.

Peggy gagged. She struggled to keep from throwing up. By the time they reached the park on Hospital Hill, she lost the battle. She flung open the passenger door and heaved.

Carlton stopped the car, which was then going no more than three miles an hour. He put it in park, shoved open his door, and stepped out. Stinky Man was gone. No one was on the trunk.

Carlton stepped away from the car. It was parked in front of the paved walk to Chimborazo Medical Museum.

After exiting the passenger side, Peggy used tissues from her purse to wipe clean her mouth and chin. She feared she had swallowed the stink and it would forever be part of her.

"Where'd he go?" she asked.

"He's dead," Carlton said. "He always dies before you get to the hospital."

"What hospital?"

"This whole hill was a tent hospital for Confederate soldiers. Thousands of them were here. Stinky Man was a soldier who had dysentery. He fell in love with a volunteer nurse. One night, he thought he might be dying. So he tried to walk to the woman's house to see her one last time. But he got lost. The story is he's trying to return to the hospital but doesn't make it before he falls over and dies."

"Well, his smell made it here," Peggy said. "You think he was a ghost? Did we just see a ghost? Why won't the smell go away?"

"It will," Carlton promised her.

And it did. In a few weeks.

He drove to Linda's house, not far from where their night had begun, with the windows down. It was five minutes before ten, and no one kissed anyone goodnight.

OTHER VIRGINIA SIGHTINGS

ABINGDON

Built in 1832, the sixty-one-room Martha Washington Inn was formerly a women's college and a hospital.

A pale and riderless ghost horse appears on the inn's south lawn. Confederate cavalry ambushed Union troops near this location in 1864. One of the wounded officers mounted his horse. When it arrived at the inn, then in use as a hospital, he was swiftly taken from his saddle and carried inside. He died that night of his wounds. No one told the horse, which waited outside for its rider to return. And waited.

The horse now returns from the afterlife, usually at night, to see if the officer is ready yet to leave the inn. So far, nay.

ALEXANDRIA

L'Ouverture Hospital, named to honor Toussaint L'Ouverture, the black liberator of Haiti, was built in 1863–64 for African-American soldiers. William Chester Minor was the surgeon there. Though excellent at his work, Minor suffered what would today be called post-traumatic stress disorder, and eventually severe delusions, from an incident when he was required by a superior officer to brand the letter D on the forehead of a Union deserter.

His ghost has returned to the hospital building but is never seen. Instead, a phantom branding iron appears. It floats in the air, business end forward. Its tip glowing red-hot, the iron lunges toward visitors to the basement, then just as quickly draws back.

The ghost isn't trying to hurt anyone. In fact, he appears to be attempting to take back the act that caused one man so much pain, and another severe mental anguish.

ARLINGTON NATIONAL CEMETERY

When doctors heal the sick, it is through the touch of nurses. A gathering of energy believed to be the helping hands of former nurses has created a powerful vortex with restorative properties on the grassy hill at the Nurses' Memorial in Arlington National Cemetery. The swirl of positive ghost energy moves between the evergreen trees and the tombstones there. Spending time near the memorial is said to recharge visitors both spiritually and physically.

Perhaps old nurses never really die, but rather continue their service from the grave.

CENTREVILLE

Built in 1854, the Old Stone Church on Braddock Road is in fine repair and continues in use as a church. That wasn't the case at the end of the War Between the States, when not much more than the walls remained. The church had to be rebuilt on the original foundation in 1872.

According to one historical account, "an inexperienced Union army" marched past the church on the way to the battlefield at Manassas. It might be pointed out, but rarely is, that the Confederate army was just as inexperienced.

After the battle, wounded Union soldiers were treated in the church.

Following Second Manassas, the area became a Confederate campground.

Today, floating balls of light are seen on the second floor of the church. They circle the room, then pass rapidly one after another through the window, as if fired from a gun.

Union sentries posted on the roof of the church at night fired shots at regular intervals to help the wounded at Manassas locate the emergency hospital. The rebuilt church appears to have a taller second story and a roof that extends above the height of that of the original church. The phantom balls of light look to be signal shots fired by a ghost who circles the room in search of a way out.

HAMPTON

The ghost of a dentist who died on the premises haunts the Hampton Dental Association offices. Employees sense the dead man's presence and have heard the sounds of a drill when no one is using it.

A clairvoyant contacted the dentist's spirit and learned he accidentally overdosed on nitrous oxide in the 1970s and had not intended to kill himself. No one knows exactly what he is drilling for. One guess is that some of the dead arrive in the afterlife with cavities.

The practice from days gone by of tying closed the mouth of the deceased before burial may have its roots in an understanding that the dead desire no sharp objects be put in their mouths.

The Jolly Roger is smiling for some reason, and this just might be it.

HAMPTON

Fort Monroe ceased military operations and became Fort Monroe National Monument in 2011. The Casement Museum, located there, houses a collection of artifacts that include nineteenth-century uniforms, weapons, and medical instruments used in the fort's hospital.

A soldier stationed at Fort Monroe shortly before it closed was arrested and detained for repeatedly firing his weapon at a ghost. After one month in confinement, the soldier was released. His first night in barracks, he fired at the ghost again. The ghost carried an amputation saw, according to the beleaguered solider, who was mustered from service after spending a second month in confinement.

His mistake wasn't in seeing a ghost. It was in thinking he could kill a person already dead.

The ghost is believed to have been a surgeon during the War Between the States. It is likely he has formed an attachment to one of the medical instruments in the Casement Museum. The saw he carries, of course, once served the opposite purpose—that of unattachment.

LEESBURG

Graydon Manor is a historic house constructed as a summer home by Washington, D.C., socialite H. B. Hibbs. The manor was later put to use as a mental-health facility.

A young woman was sent to Graydon by her parents to separate her from a wayward boyfriend. Her only mental-health issue was one of being in love.

What does a little distance matter to young lovers? Her beau visited on occasion. The girl would escape and meet him at the gazebo in the woods. Only the trees knew they were there.

Unable to convince her parents to release her from care at Graydon, the young lady over time lost the interest of her boyfriend. He stopped making the trip. Instead, he sent a letter.

It was like the limb of a tree had fallen on her heart, crushing it to pieces. Unable to endure such a cruel world, the abandoned lover hanged herself in the gazebo, leaving behind a note saying her ghost would haunt the former trysting spot until her boyfriend returned to her.

She's still hanging around. And the haunted gazebo is still standing, but with a bit of a lean of late. The structure was recently hit by a falling tree and is in a state of disrepair.

PETERSBURG

A former Confederate facility known as Howard's Grove Hospital was designated as a mental-health hospital for African-Americans in 1869. It was then called Central Lunatic Asylum. Like most state mental-health facilities, it was vastly overcrowded and underfunded.

A ghost who haunts the building wants visitors to leave the abandoned site. There's no room for even one more. The ghost will step on their toes until they're gone. The sensation of sharp pain is accompanied by no physical apparition. Some visitors have reported that the pain occurs simultaneously with a rush of frigid air up their legs.

Trespassing inside the old asylum is strictly illegal. The original structure, part of the Central State Hospital campus in Petersburg, is unsafe. Especially if you're barefoot.

PORTSMOUTH

Old Norfolk Naval Hospital, also known as Building 1 at Portsmouth Naval Medical Center, was constructed in 1827. Thousands of soldiers were treated there. Many died. One never left.

A peg-legged Confederate amputee hobbles from room to room on the top floor of the five-story hospital. The apparition audibly grunts and groans with each step. Those in the rooms below can hear his wooden leg making slow progress.

In the 1960s, according to Portsmouth Naval Medical Center historian Al Cutchin, two medical corpsmen who had heard rumors of the ghost wanted to get to the bottom of what was going on. So they conducted a ghost-hunting experiment. The corpsmen sprinkled talcum powder across the hardwood floor of a room on the fifth floor. Then they waited in the room below.

Upon hearing the thumping of a wooden leg, accompanied by the usual groans, the medics rushed upstairs to the closed room. There, they discovered alternating boot and peg prints in the otherwise undisturbed dusting of powder.

WILLIAMSBURG

The president's house at the College of William and Mary is haunted by the ghost of a French soldier whose love went up in flames inside the original structure, then called the Governor's Palace.

During the American Revolution, the mansion temporarily served as the headquarters for British general Charles Cornwallis. It was later occupied by French soldiers fighting with the Americans. Rooms there were used as a hospital, with a French surgeon in residence.

A fire burned much of the stately home in 1871, leaving only the thick outer walls intact. Everyone at the time was believed to have escaped, but it wasn't so. A local girl who was the paramour of a French soldier stayed inside the burning building rather than face the shame of her illicit tryst becoming known.

The soldier spent a life of hidden guilt. Following his death, his ghost returned to the site of his amorous liaison. It continues to inhabit the second and third floors of the current building. Perhaps this time, he is hoping to save the girl he left behind.

WEST VIRGINIA

UN-LYING EYES
DR. W. L. GRIMES DENTAL CLINIC,
1125 TWENTIETH STREET,
HUNTINGTON

TRAUMA AND SUDDEN FEAR CREATE GHOSTS.

In particular, there is something about the jarring step-by-step tumble of a body down a flight of stairs to death that is likely to create a ghost. Perhaps it is our innate fear of falling, the unanticipated loss of equilibrium, that marks such moments for decades, if not eternity. A human body is lost somewhere between its search for solid footing and its failure to fly.

It's not just scary to fall. It also hurts. Like sticks and stones, falls break bones. A body's plummet down a flight of stairs occurs in a series of bone-cracking falls. Whether backward, forward, or twisting in air, a body slams over and over again against hard, sharp angles.

In 1913, Bernice Wall left Ohio and her abusive, alcoholic husband, Cyrus, and moved to Huntington, West Virginia, in time for her five-year-old daughter, Lavina, to start school there. From time to time over the years, Lavina's father showed up at the two-story duplex Bernice rented, usually drunk and in need of money. He demanded that Bernice give him whatever cash she had on hand, the money she had earned as a waitress in town. He slung open drawers in the bedroom, strewing clothes until he found the money she had set aside for rent and groceries.

Then, as always, Cyrus Wall punished his wife for leaving him. He punished her for not having as much money as he needed.

Fear occupied the house on Twentieth Street whenever Cyrus was there. As World War I ended and America quickstepped into the new dances of the 1920s, as women won the right to vote, cut their hair short,

Photocopy of Lavina Wall's death certificate

smoked cigarettes, and wore new, loose clothes with fancy fringe and beads, his old farm truck with Ohio plates would occasionally be parked out front when Lavina and her younger sister came home from school.

When this occurred, the two girls would sit outside on the steps, hoping Cyrus would leave before they had to go inside. They spoke in whispers, if they spoke at all. When darkness fell, the two girls removed their shoes, went inside, and crept upstairs. If their mother's bedroom door was closed, they slipped into the room they shared at the top of the stairs. They closed the door as silently as possible and went to bed, trying in vain to shut out the loud curses and sounds of violence in the adjoining bedroom.

Lavina eventually finished school. A talented seamstress, she worked from home as a dressmaker. The new style of flapper dresses had by then reached the smallest towns, and everyone wanted them. The stock market boomed. Prosperity was everywhere in the 1920s. Lavina soon earned as much money as her mother. And sometimes more.

Everyone, it seemed, had money in 1929. Except for Cyrus. By the time Lavina turned twenty-one in September of that year, Cyrus had long since turned his evil intentions on her. He demanded money from Lavina, as he had from Bernice. He believed that anything the women had they owed to him, whether or not they were still his family. And Cyrus would get it with his fists, when he had to.

The women of the 1920s were far too uppity, as far as he was concerned. They shouldn't be working in the first place. They shouldn't smoke or wear loose dresses. What they should do was come back to Ohio and keep house for him. When they refused, as they did every time he asked, it was his calling as a man to knock the women down a step or two and show them where they belonged.

It wasn't wrong of Cyrus, or any man, to want his wife to come home. He'd been wanting it for more than fifteen years now. Fifteen years of failure, of violent rage fueled by poorly made bootleg liquor, drove Cyrus to visit his wife and daughters time and time again.

So it was that fear lived at the top of the stairs for Lavina Wall in October 1929. It wasn't a silent fear. It was a loud, cursing, crashing fear. A fear you could hear from across the street.

When her father's rusty farm truck pulled up outside, Lavina alerted her sister. The two of them hurried down the steep stairs in their thick autumn socks and hid just outside the back door. They listened to Cyrus lumber through the house, searching for money.

Stamping up and down the stairs, waiting for Bernice and Lavina to come home, Cyrus grew angrier minute by minute, step by step. He kicked the furniture. He slammed his hands against the walls. Soon, his rage became the clamorous heartbeat of the house.

When Lavina heard her treadle sewing machine crash to the floor, she was through hiding from the beast. He had her money now. It had been hidden in the little, tilting tool drawer of her beloved sewing machine. Lavina's livelihood depended on that machine, and it was as surely broken as was her heart.

For once, she was going to do something about the dark evil trampling her life to bits. She would tolerate her abusive father's thefts and threats no longer. Lavina told her sister to stay outside.

Since Cyrus had her money, maybe he would turn tail and leave if she screamed at him. Maybe he'd be gone by the time her mother came home.

Her face scalded with tears, Lavina took a deep breath and went inside the house with the determined purpose to stand up for herself. And for her mother and sister. She marched to the bottom of the stairs.

"Enough!" she yelled. Her body trembled with anger and fear. But her voice didn't. It was loud and clear. "Go home! No one wants you here!"

Cyrus appeared at the top of the stairs. Her father, long since estranged from her heart, swayed in drunken disorder. He leaned his back against the wall to steady himself, smiling from ear to ear.

He carried her money in his fists. His right hand clutched three five-dollar bills and one two-dollar bill in a tight roll, the way Lavina had hidden it. From between the finger and thumb of his left hand, a gleaming twenty-dollar gold piece bounced light from the landing window as Cyrus held it up for his daughter to view. The coin was his trophy, the shining emblem of his dominance over her.

Thirty-seven dollars represented more than a month's work for Lavina. She needed to buy material with that money. She needed to eat. For Cyrus, the money meant he could stay drunk for another month without a lick of work on his part. He was the king of his house, and he was the king of theirs. Lavina's labor and dreams meant nothing to him. Nor did her mother's. He mattered, they didn't.

Cyrus laughed when he saw his daughter's face streaked with tears. The girl could barely breathe. He laughed and wouldn't stop laughing. He was laughing still when she reached the top of the stairs and wildly swung her arms at him. She slapped her hands through the air as rapidly as she knew how, hoping they landed anywhere that might make him stop laughing.

Lavina, even at twenty-one, was a wisp of a girl. Slender from top to bottom, she weighed no more than a hundred pounds. Cyrus pushed her. He laughed louder when she lost her balance, flailing her hands, falling backward. He could have reached out to steady her, but his hands were busy holding tight the money he'd stolen.

For both of them, what happened next was in slow motion.

Unable to brace herself, Lavina dropped down the stairs. Twisting to avoid the repeated shock and pain of hitting the risers, Lavina sprawled at the bottom of the steps. Her face pressed the hardwood floor of the living room. Her legs were turned at odd angles, somewhere above and behind her, still on the stairs.

Blinding pain raced through her back, where she'd first slammed the edge of a riser. Lavina struggled to keep her eyes open to prove to herself that she wasn't dead. When she breathed, it burned like fire. Her ribs were cracked. Maybe something worse. One eye slowly closed, swelling shut above her badly bruised cheek. It felt to Lavina as if she'd been hit in the face by a baseball bat. But her back hurt worse.

Cyrus watched his daughter for a minute. He saw her hand move. He pocketed his cash and came downstairs, still smiling.

He could easily have picked her up and carried her in his arms. Cyrus, though, was none too steady on his feet at the moment. He made Lavina's younger sister help.

"Grab hold of anything," he said. "She's passed out now."

The two managed to hoist Lavina upstairs. They placed her in bed, where she would stay for almost two weeks. By the time Bernice brought her daughter to the local hospital, at the insistence of a physician who visited Lavina in the home, it was too late to save her life.

Most ghosts of accidents haunt the locations where they suffered the violent mishaps that results in their deaths. They tend to relive the accidents over and over. Yet it was Lavina's fate to linger in pain for weeks. For reasons of her own, she lingers still. Her apparition continues to haunt the house, as does her father's violent anger. His rage lives on as a dark cloud of fear at the top of the stairs.

In 1973, Huntington dentist William L. Grimes and his father purchased the property and began remodeling the two-story duplex as a dental office and clinic. Soon after the work was completed, Dr. Grimes and his father opened their new practice. Dr. Grimes said he first noticed the presence of a ghost while he and his dad were remodeling.

"But I didn't see Lavina until 1975," he said, "and then only in brief flashes."

Instead of being concerned about seeing a ghost, Dr. Grimes was fascinated by what the ghost was seeing. There was something about her eyes.

He described Lavina as a slight figure with long black hair. She was so slight, in fact, that he believed the girl to be no more than twelve years old. He saw her so often those early years that he became enchanted by her ghost. He painted her picture. The portrait hangs today in his dental practice at 1125 Twentieth Street in Huntington.

"She continually appeared to me as I was wallpapering the stairwell, just quick flashes every time," Dr. Grimes said.

He felt like the ghost he now calls Livy was trying to communicate with him that she was a victim who had been hurt. He saw her most often in a doorway near the bottom of the stairs.

"I could see Livy, but I couldn't hear her," he said. "She was trying to express her emotions with her eyes. That is why her eyes are so sad in the portrait I painted. I couldn't get those sad eyes out of my mind. I definitely lost my fear of her. I just wanted to help her."

In the painting, Lavina's gaze is directed upward. Her dark eyes are large and haunting—as haunting as the feeling of fear that languishes still at the top of the stairs.

One of Dr. Grimes's former assistants said in a recent television interview that she felt a persistent presence at the top of the stairs. When she climbed the steps to the former bedroom where Dr. Grimes maintains his patient files, it was like entering a cloud of palpable fear. It was a fear that felt like a weight, a darkness that surrounded her and held her in place, an ominous pressure that encased her body. It was Lavina's fear of her father.

The fear at the top of the stairs soon became the assistant's own.

"It got to where I just couldn't go up there any longer," the assistant said. "Someone else had to do the filing."

A psychic who investigated the haunting at Dr. Grimes's invitation said she heard derisive, drunken laughter while standing on the landing. A man's laughter. The psychic also experienced visions of a dark-haired girl sprawled face down at the bottom of the stairs. The girl's arms and legs are askew, she said. The girl appeared to be writhing in pain.

But the ghost doesn't exist falling down the stairs. Neither does it exist as a figure sprawled at the bottom steps. Nor is Lavina a ghost lying on her deathbed. Lavina stands in the ground-floor doorway, looking up. Her purpose isn't to relive her death. It is something else.

The 1929 death certificate of Lavina Wall lists her cause of death as something rather curious for someone who took a bad spill. Indeed, it contains no mention of her falling down the stairs. Her fall, however, is not conjecture. An early newspaper account of her death, based on information provided by her mother, stated that Lavina died of complications from a fall down the stairs in her home two weeks prior to the date of her final breath, which came at three in the morning on October 28.

No autopsy was performed. Dr. John Keesee, who first treated Lavina in her home on October 20 for injuries from her fall, noted that, upon death, the inside of Lavina's mouth and throat were reddened and blistered by burning. The doctor stated her cause of death as acute gastroenteritis. He further noted with a question mark that a contributory factor might have been "Liquor Poisoning."

At first glance, gastroenteritis seems an unlikely cause of death for a young woman who was pushed backward down the stairs. Whether or not Lavina suffered internal injuries from the fall is unproven. But it was documented that she experienced dire pain and distress from the moment of the fall until her death two weeks later.

Why would our slender girl's mouth and throat be burned, and why would liquor poisoning be a suspected contributory factor in her death? The answer is Prohibition.

Booze, simply put, was a standard home remedy for pain. Because the prohibition of the sale of liquor was in force in the United States from 1919 to 1933, potable liquor was not available for consumption at the time of Lavina's injuries. Distasteful and damaging chemicals were, by government decree, added during those years to over-the-counter products, such as cologne and hair tonic, that contained enough alcohol to induce people to consume them to achieve the same effect as drinking liquor.

It was a known practice of those who wanted to drink during Prohibition, and who could find no other source, to strain over-the-counter products high in alcohol through a loaf of bread. This was believed to make chemically treated alcohol products safe to drink. It didn't.

Illegal hooch carried a similar risk. The 1920s saw an increasingly common cause of death and disability caused by bootleggers' products. Many stills used lead coils or lead soldering, which gave off acetate of lead, a dangerous poison. Some bootleggers used recipes that included iodine, creosote, or even embalming fluid.

Lavina's slow extraction from this life was certainly not painless. The psychic who visited Dr. Grimes's dental practice insisted that the girl she saw sprawled on the floor had suffered a broken back.

What mother could see her daughter in pain and not do something about it? Lavina's burned mouth and throat are clear evidence that she was given copious amounts of chemically treated or haphazardly poisoned alcohol as a pain reliever. Lavina's pain did not subside over those two remaining weeks, and it is left for one to assume she spent many hours passed out from alcohol consumption.

In her portrait as a ghost, Lavina's mouth is conspicuously closed. Since her mouth and throat were severely burned the last days of her life, it is likely that she was unable to speak. She thus tells her story not with words, but with her presence.

The reason Lavina chooses to stay in her house a hundred years after she and her mother moved there is in her eyes in the portrait Dr. Grimes painted. She is by all accounts a quiet ghost. Her stare, however, is another story. It's a stare of accusation.

Her eyes scream bloody murder.

Lavina Wall was killed one way and died another. Her death certificate didn't get to the bottom of her cause of death. The purpose of Lavina's haunting is to identify the true cause of her death. Her purpose is to accuse her father of the act that eventually killed her. Lavina wants the world to know the truth. Lavina's ghost seeks justice.

Her large, haunting eyes trap her father and hold him in place at the top of the stairs. Her intense stare pins him there like a moth on a specimen board, like a photo of someone wanted for murder pinned to the bulletin board at the post office.

In truth, Lavina was pushed to her death down those hardwood steps.

It is a coincidence of history that Lavina Wall wasn't the only entity to fall that autumn. So did prosperity. The day after Lavina died, the Roaring Twenties came to a screeching halt with the devastating October 29, 1929, crash of the stock market known as Black Tuesday.

Dr. Grimes says most of his patients don't mind a ghost making his dental clinic her earthly home. Patients can view her closed-mouth portrait in his office even today. Livy, according to Dr. Grimes, belongs there as much as anyone, although he admits most of the people he sees in his practice eventually open their mouths.

THE BEAT GOES ON
WEIRTON MEDICAL CENTER,
601 COLLIERS WAY,
WEIRTON

OF THE NUMEROUS PHYSICAL ITEMS that have been documented to hold the spirit of a ghost, perhaps none is as startling as the haunting at Weirton Medical Center. The ghost of a patient makes his presence known by sound alone. He is a ghost you can hear. But he never says a word.

Not long ago, a member of the housekeeping department was preparing to buff the floor of an unoccupied room on the fifth-floor cardiac-care unit. The housekeeper noticed that a heart monitor in the room was beeping. At first, it didn't bother him. It is common for a heart monitor to beep when not in use as a signal that it has been left turned on. This monitor, however, seemed to have a pulse of its own. It was registering the rhythm of a normal heartbeat, as if still attached to a patient.

The housekeeper felt a chill trace the outline of his spine to the back of his neck. He stopped working. He stared at the monitor, willing it to stop. But it continued to emit the perpetual beeps of a living human heart. *Beep-beep, beep-beep, beep-beep.*

When he could stand it no longer, the floor tech left the room and approached the nursing station. A night nurse smiled knowingly when he told her the monitor was registering the normal activity of a human heart when no one was in the room.

She returned with the floor tech to the room to remove the heart monitor. The machine, he now saw, was not plugged in, and hadn't been.

She explained that the particular heart monitor wasn't the problem. Any heart monitor left unattended in that room, she told him, had a tendency to come on by itself. She further noted that most of the nursing staff in the cardiac-care unit knew not to leave a monitor in the room when it was unoccupied.

A heart monitor in a hospital setting is, of course, the standard signal of when life becomes death. As life leaves a body, the heart stops. The spirit lingers awhile yet. We know there is a window of time between dying and the possibility of being revived. Many people have been dead for moments, or even several minutes, and have been brought back to life.

Perhaps one patient who passed on at Weirton Medical Center believes he won't have to be dead as long as his heart monitor sounds the activity of a beating heart. Though bodily dead, the patient's spirit appears to have retained a pulse. *Beep-beep, beep-beep, beep-beep.*

It is up to neither us nor the science of medicine to determine when a person has given up the ghost and is irretrievably dead. It's up to the ghost. And it remains the ghost's decision when to move on to the other side. Or not.

What we can be sure of is that, for one former patient at Weirton Medical Center, home is indeed where the heart is.

KLEPTO GHOST
TRANS-ALLEGHENY INSANE ASYLUM, 71 ASYLUM DRIVE, WESTON

THE GHOST OF A GIRL NAMED NANCY wanders the buildings and grounds of the massive Trans-Allegheny Insane Asylum, located off West Second Street in Weston, West Virginia. The state asylum, closed in 1994, is quite an impressive structure, one inside of which a young girl could easily become lost. But Nancy isn't lost. Something else is.

Someone at Trans-Allegheny stole her heart.

Trans-Allegheny was designed in the 1850s. Construction of the Gothic Revival structure, which resembles a forbidding castle, was completed soon after the War Between the States. The main building, with its distinctive green and white clock tower, has been designated a National Historic Landmark and is noted as the second-largest hand-cut stone building in the world. The largest is the Kremlin in Moscow.

Trans-Allegheny is one of those buildings as scary on the inside as it is ominous on the outside. Chains attached to walls, human cages, straitjackets, electroshock therapy so powerful it sometimes broke bones, and lobotomies were employed to treat everything from daydreaming to mania. All are part of the sad history of the treatment of mental disorders in the United States.

After the admission of the first patient in 1864, thousands of people were committed to living out nightmare existences within the stone walls of Trans-Allegheny Insane Asylum. Many patients were impaired by severe mental disabilities. Some had birth defects. Many were committed for moral transgressions including marital infidelity and atheism. An overzealous obsession with one's hobby would suffice. Any habit your family or community found socially repugnant might have landed you in

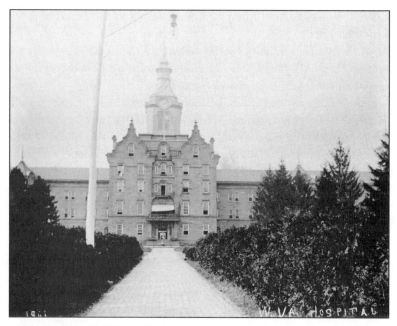

Historic photograph of Trans-Allegheny Lunatic Asylum in Weston, West Virginia,
later called Weston State Hospital.
WEST VIRGINIA STATE ARCHIVES

the asylum. Heaven forbid you should develop a nervous facial tic or find yourself routinely laughing out loud in situations others didn't find funny.

As an added indignity, Trans-Allegheny was for most of its history understaffed and vastly overcrowded. Originally designed to house 250 patients, the facility routinely held in excess of 2,000. In an independent investigation conducted in 1949, it was found to be housing more than 2,400 patients. Lobotomies were routinely and crudely performed, and unruly patients were still being locked in cages, according to articles in the *Charleston Gazette*.

While some patients suffered from the misunderstanding of mental disorders and treatments now considered abuse, or even torture, others suffered simple neglect. Many endured assaults at the hands of other mental patients.

Although Nancy did not suffer violence at the hands of another patient at Trans-Allegheny, she was indeed a victim of another patient's mental imbalance. She was the victim of theft.

Among the myriad reasons people were routinely placed in mental hospitals was kleptomania. While getting caught stealing money or things of value would have sent a person to jail, stealing things of little or no monetary value might have earned him or her a room in an insane asylum. At the time of Trans-Allegheny's closing, it is estimated that 5 to 10 percent of its population had been diagnosed with kleptomania.

In Nancy's day, patients in mental institutions were allowed to bring along only a few personal items. Nancy wore a bracelet, a simple chain with a single heart-shaped charm. Her father is said to have given it to her on her twelfth birthday. The heart for Nancy was a symbol of love. She treasured it.

She kept the bracelet in the drawer of a metal bedside stand when she slept. One morning, it was gone.

Nancy was inconsolable. She would not be comforted until her bracelet was found and returned. The staff allowed the girl to take short outings to look for her stolen heart. She walked the grounds of Trans-Allegheny with her head down. Inside the facility, she stared at other patients to see if one might be wearing her bracelet. She sneaked out of her room at night in bedclothes and wandered the halls on the third floor, peeking into other patients' rooms.

She never found her bracelet. By all accounts, she is still looking for it. Her search did not end with death. Nancy has returned to Trans-Allegheny from beyond her physical life to look for her missing heart. It appears she's staying until she finds it.

Along with the grounds, a portion of Trans-Allegheny Lunatic Asylum remains open as a historical site. The facility's turbulent history has led to several hauntings, according to the current owners and various witnesses. Numerous ghosts continue to be reported inside the massive stone building. A spiral staircase to abandoned patient rooms on the third floor awakens with the sound of whispering voices and the laughter of children, but only when there are living human footfalls upon the steps. A disembodied voice saying "Go home" was recently documented during a visit by a team of researchers for the television series *Ghost Hunters*. Some who have toured the abandoned asylum report being touched by unseen entities in a section where patients, often in restraints, were held in isolation. The owners provide regularly scheduled tours for ghost hunters.

Visitors to the grounds at night have seen Nancy's face peering from a third-floor window. Others inside the building have looked outside to capture glimpses of a female ghost walking the grounds, head down, hair covering her face. Nancy also appears at times as a girl-shaped shadow moving silently across the walls of the hallways on the third floor of the main building.

Nancy is a searching ghost, and it seems her situation may be hopeless.

From dozens, if not hundreds, of examples, we know that ghosts attach themselves to favored objects. A portrait on the wall, an old, comfortable chair, an antique bed—all have been known to hold ghosts for years, decades, and perhaps forever. Even the smallest things may travel the years in company with a human ghost.

Unlike ghosts who are attached to particular places, ghosts attached to items go where the items go. An otherworldly attachment to an artifact from life can become a passport for ghost travel. When you buy an antique pocket watch or a wedding ring online from a shop overseas, it may bring with it a come-along ghost with a foreign accent.

Nancy's situation is different. Her ghost is attached to an item she cannot find.

We don't know what behavioral problems brought Nancy to Trans-Allegheny at such a young age. We don't know how long she was there, if she was incarcerated until her death, or if she was released, got married, had children, and died elsewhere. What we do know is that Nancy is back, trapped at the time of her original loss, and she won't leave.

A large tree on the grounds of Trans-Allegheny has been dubbed "the Klepto Tree." It shades the southeast corner of the property in the vicinity of where Nancy's ghost is most often seen when she appears outside the main building.

"A patient who suffered from kleptomania stole things from all over the place and buried them," Rebecca Jordan Gleason said in a recent interview. Gleason is the co-owner and operations manager of Trans-Allegheny. She believes Nancy's stolen bracelet might be nearby.

With that in mind, Gleason hosted television treasure hunters George Wyant and Tim Saylor on a visit to Trans-Allegheny to search the grounds with metal detectors. Their search was broadcast as an episode of the National Geographic Channel reality series *Diggers* on August 28, 2013.

In a day's work, the treasure hunters uncovered a number of historical artifacts. They also unearthed a small horde of inexpensive personal items, including jewelry, buried as a single cache under the Klepto Tree.

Evidently, Nancy's bracelet was not among the kleptomaniac's stolen loot. Her ghost continues to walk the halls and grounds of Trans-Allegheny. The bracelet may be hidden elsewhere. Perhaps it will never be found. One thing, though, can be counted upon. Nancy will not stop looking.

Searching ghosts are attached to physical items that remain behind. A ghost seeking the precious artifact of its earthly existence continues to search until the item is, if ever, found. In eternity, the passage of decades is of no concern.

OTHER WEST VIRGINIA SIGHTINGS

BECKLEY

Jackie Withrow Hospital, formerly Pinecrest Hospital, opened in 1930 as a tuberculosis sanatorium. Since 1970, it has provided long-term care for the elderly. The hospital, located at 105 South Eisenhower Drive, is owned and managed by the state of West Virginia.

In days gone by, a large number of patients who succumbed to tuberculosis were cremated at the facility. This resulted in a regularly occurring foul odor from the crematorium smokestack. The stink of burning flesh was said to be especially bad in the summer months. Since the facility operated for decades without air conditioning, windows were kept open on warm nights, meaning that the odor permeated the rooms. Current hauntings include the ghost of a young girl who, carrying lilacs, floats through the halls either late at night or early in the morning. Patients and visitors alike have reported a strong scent of lilacs accompanying the apparition. The pleasing scent is said to linger for hours. The ghost has been nicknamed "the Flower Girl."

Another ghost has long been reported at the hospital. An elderly woman in a blue dress with her hair in a bun is seemingly an original haunting from the years when the facility was known as Pinecrest. "The Bun Lady" is believed to have been a volunteer nurse's aide. She appears only at night in various hospital rooms. Holding a box of matches, she hovers over sleeping patients. The Bun Lady appears to be a specific type of messenger ghost who functions as a harbinger of death.

CHARLESTON

The ghost of a woman in a fur coat covered with blood haunts the area just outside the emergency-room entrance at Charleston Area Medical Center, located at 501 Morris Street. Known as "Aunt Blood," the ghost reportedly resembles Aunt Bee from the old *Andy Griffith Show*.

Apparently unaware of her appearance, the blood-spattered ghost rushes to aid accident victims with her arms wide open. It is believed Aunt Blood's intention is to comfort the injured as they are wheeled into the hospital for emergency care.

DENMAR

The State Colored Tuberculosis Sanatorium in the remote, unincorporated community of Denmar, West Virginia, admitted its first patient in 1919 and closed in 1990. The facility is operated today as a medium-security correctional institution. A birthing center for federal prisoners occupies the original nurses' quarters, while a ghost who refuses to accept his death continues showing up for work in the main building.

Described as a short African-American doctor in a white lab coat with a stethoscope around his neck, the ghost doctor steps off the elevator in the morning. He nods and smiles to whomever is present, as if to say good morning, then promptly fades away.

A ghost of habit, the dedicated doctor repeats his lifetime ritual. For some hardworking souls, death is not cause enough for taking a sick day.

HUNTINGTON

Once known as the Hospital for Incurables, the renovated state mental hospital at 1530 Norway Avenue in Huntington, West Virginia, now operates as Mildred Mitchell-Bateman Hospital, a psychiatric-care facility and training site for health-care professionals. The original hospital was noted in the 1940s and 1950s for severe overcrowding and outdated facilities. According to a report in the *Huntington Herald-Advertiser*, the children's ward was accessible only by climbing "three flights of narrow steel stairs, so twisting and turning that it is almost impossible to carry anything, or anybody up or down."

Fourteen patients, all female, died in a fire at the hospital one November night in 1952. Five were under the age of sixteen. The oldest was Ada Carver, who was eighty-nine, while the youngest was Lena Wentz, age eleven.

Among other recurring sightings, the shadowy apparition of a young female ghost is seen in the evening hours. She holds the hand of an old woman, patiently leading her to the hospital morgue. It is believed that those who follow the ghostly duo into the morgue will not return.

MILTON

Morris Memorial Hospital, on Morris Memorial Road in Milton, West Virginia, opened its doors in 1936 as a residential hospital for children with polio. In later years, the facility saw use as a nursing home. Now abandoned by the living, the site is haunted by a small number of ghosts who have chosen to extend their hospital stay. They are most often experienced as the echoing sounds of laughter in the portion of the original building used as a school.

Local legend suggests that one of the teachers was a talented jokester and a master of the unexpected punch line. Moments of glee were likely rare occurrences in the lives of children suffering the crippling effects of infantile paralysis and separated from their peers attending normal schools.

Happy ghosts are not as common as ghosts saddened by sudden or violent deaths, traumatic life events, and disturbed or improper burials. But some blithe spirits do return to revisit happy moments of their lives.

MOUNDSVILLE

The West Virginia State Penitentiary on Jefferson Avenue in Moundsville looks like a stone castle, complete with turrets and battlements, walls five feet thick, and a central tower section more than six hundred feet across. In operation from 1876 to 1995, the prison housed a notoriously violent population. Its hospital and accompanying morgue saw heavy duty over the years. The bodies of ninety-four executed prisoners were brought to the hospital for medical verification of death. The majority of executions were by hanging, and in later years by a brief visit to the prison electric chair, known as "Old Sparky."

Numerous hauntings have been documented at the prison. None is perhaps as dramatic as the ghostly apparition of inmate Frank Hyer, who was hanged at the end of a twenty-foot drop on June 19, 1931. Frank's hanging was conducted at a time when the public was allowed to view prison executions. The events were so popular among local citizens as to be known as "Moundsville Picnics."

It was certainly no picnic for Frank. He was hanged so efficiently that his head popped off when the noose tightened at the end of his drop. His head and body were rushed to the prison hospital, where both were pronounced dead.

Frank had no choice but to bodily leave this world. His headless ghost, however, is of a different mind and has decided to hang around the prison. Frank is seen in brief flashes in various locations throughout the facility.

Public tours of the historic prison are available April through November.

PARKERSBURG

When Anne Camden passed away in 1918, she left the family mansion in Parkersburg, West Virginia, to the city, to be used as a hospital. Soon known as Camden Clark Memorial Hospital, the original 104-bed facility has since seen many improvements, including the addition of a three-story patient wing in 1936. The next year, Ella Bloomhart was named director of nursing.

Although Ella has been dead many years now, she continues to visit patients in the east wing of Camden Clark. Ella's ghost is most often seen wearing an outdated nurse's uniform. She goes about her business without speaking to anyone, entirely focused on providing care to the extent that she occasionally walks through walls to gain access to patient rooms.

WHEELING

A shadow person is seen with some regularity at the REM West Virginia Intermediate Care nursing facility, located on Greggson, Clinton & Potomac Road in Wheeling. Known to staff and patients alike as "the Shadow Guy," he is often seen wearing a striped shirt.

Boasting the ability to move rapidly across rooms, shadow people rank among the scariest ghostly apparitions. Usually associated with a particular item of clothing, often a hat, a shadow person is an adult-sized ghost who appears as a three-dimensional shadow with no discernible facial features. It does not reflect light. A shadow person may stand perfectly still for extended periods of time, seemingly to avoid having its presence detected. Once detected, however, it moves quickly to find a new hiding spot in the darker reaches of a room or building. The shadow appears to drop to the floor, race across open space, and disappear into existing shadows such as those in an open closet or under a bed, where it waits.

Seemingly without personality or purpose, shadow people appear to be ghosts who live in fear of discovery. They are watchers and are not known to pose a physical threat to the living. What circumstances create shadow people is a topic of lively debate among paranormal researchers. One popular theory purports that shadow people are time travelers who become stuck in the past and are waiting for their bodies to materialize in the future time and place where they originated their travel. In this sense, shadow people may be considered ghosts of the living. And if they are indeed time travelers, shadow people may be the ghosts of people not yet born.

The shadow ghost wearing a striped shirt at the Wheeling nursing facility is likely trying to get along with the living and is troubled by the terror he instills in people when they see him.